A STROKE OF LUCK

A STROKE OF LUCK

Music, Medicine, and a Miraculous Recovery

D. Bruce Hughes

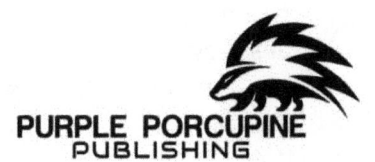

PURPLE PORCUPINE
PUBLISHING

Copyright © 2025 D. Bruce Hughes

All rights reserved. No part of this book may be reproduced, stored or transmitted in any form or by any means, electronic, mechanical, photocopying, recording, scanning and/or otherwise used in any manner for the purposes of training artificial intelligence technologies without written permission from the publisher.

Under no circumstances will any legal responsibility or blame be held against the publisher and or author for any reparation, damages, or monetary loss due to the information herein, either directly or indirectly.

Purple Porcupine Publishing
P.O. Box 555, Stewiacke, NS B0N 2J0
Purpleporcupine.ca

Editor: Penelope Jackson
Foreword: Jake Swan, MD

Library and Archives Canada Cataloguing in Publication

Title: A stroke of luck : music, medicine, and a miraculous recovery / D. Bruce Hughes ; foreword by Jake Swan, MD.
Names: Hughes, D. Bruce, author.
Description: First edition.
Identifiers: Canadiana (print) 20240514475 | Canadiana (ebook) 2024051825X | ISBN 9781738899555
   (softcover) | ISBN 9781738899562 (EPUB)
Subjects: LCSH: Hughes, D. Bruce—Health. | LCSH: Guitarists—New Brunswick—Biography. | LCSH: Rock
  musicians—New Brunswick—Biography. | LCSH: Cerebrovascular disease—Patients—Biography. | LCGFT:
  Autobiographies.
Classification: LCC ML419.H893 A3 2025 | DDC 787.87166092—dc23

To my wife, Monica, and our dog, Willow.

To all the healthcare workers that saved me and gave me a second chance at life, especially Dr. Bouma, Dr. Archer, and Dr. Swan, and the 3NE Stroke Rehab team at Dr. Everett Chalmers Hospital.

To all the stroke survivors and their families I have met on my journey.

To my friend Linda Robinson for help me get this story told.

To my bandmates.

TABLE OF CONTENTS

FOREWORD IX

INTRODUCTION XIII

CHAPTER ONE - THE STROKES 1

CHAPTER TWO - THE EARLY DAYS 11

CHAPTER THREE - LEARNING SELF-ADVOCACY 34

CHAPTER FOUR - MAKING PROGRESS 51

CHAPTER FIVE - HOMEWARD BOUND 70

CHAPTER SIX - BACK TO MUSIC 82

CHAPTER SEVEN - BRUCE HUGHES SHOULD HAVE DIED 98

CHAPTER EIGHT - A LONG WINTER 107

CHAPTER NINE - DAD 126

CHAPTER TEN - MORE MUSIC 147

EPILOGUE 177

ABOUT THE AUTHOR 180

AUTHOR'S NOTE 182

Foreword

After successfully arguing that our Interventional Radiology group had a moral obligation to take on endovascular thrombectomy for acute stroke patients in New Brunswick, Brian Archer thumbtacked a copy of a help-wanted ad to the wall of our reporting room. The original had supposedly been posted in the London *Times* by famed Arctic explorer Ernest Shackleton.

MEN WANTED
For hazardous journey, low wages,
bitter cold, long hours of complete darkness,
safe return doubtful. Honour and recognition
in event of success.

Brian championed the treatment, and Darren Ferguson and John Whelan, two other interventional radiologists in our department, quickly took up the cause. I, being more of the cowardly lion of our group, shuddered at the sensation of dragging an open metal stent through the delicate vessels of the brain, knowing I might traumatize the tissue-paper-like endothelium and that at any moment, I could do irreparable damage to some unlucky person's thinking centre. When you treat acute strokes, people die on the table. Sometimes they make it out of your department and die a few days or weeks later.

The lesson that took me the longest to learn was that if you don't treat strokes, people also die. More of them die. More of them end up with permanent disability. And the disabilities they suffer are more severe. Despite all the things that can go wrong, and despite the internalized doubts of the operator, bare, pragmatic statistics bear out the fact that, under the right circumstances, if you are having a stroke, an interventional radiologist should try to wiggle their way up your vascular system and attempt to suck out the blood clot in the blocked artery.

Still, there are limits. When a middle cerebral artery has been blocked for too long, we won't attempt to open it. When we've made multiple attempts and can't get the vessel open, we sometimes have to abandon ship to avoid causing a massive intracranial hemorrhage.

But there is a special case when we will go hell-for-leather to get a blood vessel open. Bruce was such a case.

The basilar artery supplies blood to your brain stem. The brain stem is the hub that connects all your higher brain function to the rest of your body. If a housefly lands on your cheek, your sensory nerves tell your brain about the tickling sensation on your face, you process the information by some sort of magic, the understanding of which is well outside my pay grade, and then your motor cortex sends a signal to the nerves in your arms and hand, via tracts through the brain stem and spinal cord, to brush the fly away.

If a blood clot settles in the basilar artery and deprives those hub-neurons of oxygen, suddenly the signals have nowhere to go. The housefly can set up shop in your nostril, and there's really nothing you can do about it.

While patients with an untreated brain stem stroke will often simply die (after all, the signals from your brain instructing your heart how to beat and your diaphragm to breath may be severed), occasionally these patients can end up in a permanent state of being "locked in," in which they can perceive the world, and can process it, but cannot react to it or communicate. *Locked In Locked Out* by Dr. Shawn Jennings is a firsthand account of this harrowing condition. While Dr. Jennings is an inspirational optimist and shows us that there certainly is a purposeful life to be lived after suffering such a devastating medical insult, it is nonetheless our moral duty to go to the ends of the earth to at least attempt to dampen the effects of these particular strokes.

The juvenile grandiosity of excited young medical students often lends itself to thoughts like "Maybe I'll save the person who cures cancer!" (Not so much thought about is "What if I accidentally save the next Hitler?" but that's a topic for another day.) Unbelievable as it seems, thanks to providence, and to the mentorship and kindness of Brian Archer, I have had the enormous privilege of being a small cog in the machine that saved Bruce—a man who is doing more for stroke care than I could ever dream of doing.

While that Shackleton "Men Wanted" ad may have been a little hyperbolic, stroke care does take a toll on its providers.

Drs. Archer and Whelan have left the building, so to speak. And while Dr. Ferguson is still going strong, I, myself, am contemplating a career change in the interest of my own health. Thankfully a new crop of dedicated (and in my case, much better skilled) New Brunswick interventional radiologists have risen to the occasion. Drs. Meagher, Salgado, and Dunn have taken up the torch. We can always use more, though. And while safe return may be doubtful, acute stroke care promises one hell of a voyage.

Jake Swan, MD

Introduction

My name is Bruce Hughes, but some people now call me the "Miracle Man" because of something that happened to me at the age of fifty-eight, something that changed my life forever.

I was a semi-retired youth advocate and a musician living in the picturesque community of Upper Keswick, near Fredericton, New Brunswick. On Wednesday, May 11, 2017, I had a wonderful day of celebration, not knowing what was waiting for me in the coming weeks—events that would turn my life upside down and threaten my very existence.

I was marking my wedding anniversary with Monica, the woman I have loved for thirty-six years. The year leading up to this point had been very tough for both of us and we desperately needed some lightness.

While hiking to a waterfall nine months earlier, Monica fell and was laid up for two months with a broken arm, hand, and thumb. When she finally returned to work, she only lasted a few days before she broke her back in a serious car accident courtesy of a texting driver. Monica required full home care, which I did my best to provide for seven months. I was exhausted from caring for her and we were both frustrated with how long the healing process was taking.

In addition to it being our anniversary, it was media day for Fredericton's largest local music event, the Harvest Jazz and Blues Festival held every year in September. The HJBF is not only highly acclaimed locally but also draws musicians and music lovers nationally and internationally. The Blind Dog, a band I played in for many years and with whom I had made numerous HJBF appearances, was going to be playing a reunion show that year, after an eighteen-year hiatus. I sat along with other band members and fans in Dolan's Pub waiting for the announcement of our appearance, which was enthusiastically received by the full house at the pub.

Our local newspaper, *The Daily Gleaner*, interviewed me about the reunion show. The reporter, Adam Bowie, wasn't around when we used to play, so he wanted to know more about us. He was a good reporter with a keen interest in the music scene. I looked forward to reading his article in the newspaper the following day.

Even after all those years, the acknowledgments created a nice little buzz. I was honoured that our band was recognized for our contribution to the music scene all those years ago and that we were asked to bring the band back again. Admittedly, it was also good to have a few hours free from the caregiving responsibilities at home. It was a good distraction, a "mental health day."

With something else to focus on for the next four months, caring for my wife became a little easier, even though timelines were getting tighter. I had to schedule rehearsals, find a venue, select songs, and keep in contact with former band members who were going to perform. But music was always something that made me smile and gave me a euphoric feeling. It was a much-needed slice of happiness at a time when there was a lot of hurt.

That joyful feeling lasted about three weeks. Then, in a heartbeat, it disappeared.

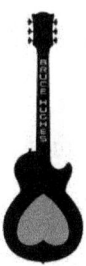

Chapter One

The Strokes

The last couple of days of May saw me feeling run down, dragging my ass around the house, just not myself. I thought maybe I was coming down with the flu, a cold; maybe my allergies were getting worse or I had an inner ear infection. Who knew? I surely didn't. My neck was sore, but that wasn't uncommon. I was the victim of a car accident in 1986 and it's left me with chronic pain in my back and neck. I tried to ride it out on my couch at night. Monica and I each had a couch in the living room, and she slept upstairs. I was determined not to give my symptoms to Monica, not wanting to add to her misery. She'd been through enough in the last year—surely I could deal with this shitty feeling of the past few days and keep it from her.

Early on the morning of May 31, we were on our couches, and I told her I still wasn't feeling well. She had a doctor's appointment the next day, and since she hadn't driven since her accident, I suggested she try to drive to the community mailbox just up the road to see if she could possibly drive herself the next day, in case I couldn't. She was starting to be able to walk a little, but driving could put too much strain on her back. I really hoped she could drive again. I needed a break and time to heal myself.

About 8:30 a.m., I went to get up from my couch to check my computer for any messages I may have missed the last couple of days. Monica was in the kitchen putting on the kettle for our coffee. Our dog, Willow, was all over me, anxious for some exercise, I thought, due to our inability to even walk her lately.

As soon as I got to my feet—BAM! Staggering to the left, unable to get my balance, my right arm tingling, I started sweating profusely, having a hard time answering my terrified wife's question: "Do you want me to call 911?"

Now on the floor, stunned and shocked by what was happening, I said a garbled yes, and she made the call. Monica was so worried but kept it together as she talked with the operator on the other end, giving them our address and describing my symptoms. We luckily live a short distance from an ambulance bay in our rural region of Keswick Valley, so in no time I could hear the siren approaching, echoing through the river valley like we'd heard so many times before. This time was different only because we knew where they were headed. Oddly comforting.

In the next instant, the feelings of numbness and disorientation and my slurred speech all disappeared. I sat up, feeling better than I had in days, as if nothing had happened or I had recovered from what ailed me. I didn't know what to think, and Monica didn't either. It made zero sense.

Within the next minute, the ambulance arrived and entered via the front door to our sunporch, where the two male paramedics quickly took the info from my wife and me, tested all my vitals, and within half an hour proclaimed that everything appeared normal, even though we all thought I had earlier presented like I was having a stroke. They were as dumbfounded as I was and suggested I go to the emergency room at the Dr. Everett Chalmers Hospital in Fredericton, a half hour away, to get checked out to be sure. I could go with them or on my own, but I should go. Good advice I was certain to take.

Since I had been on the couch for a couple of days, I decided I would like to have a shower and shave, then go get checked out at the hospital. So, I signed off their release form and sent the ambulance on its way.

Monica and I figured that while I was showering she should take Willow for a walk, before we went to the hospital. She was wound from all the inactivity recently and today's drama didn't help, so out the door they went and I headed upstairs to the bathroom.

Within a minute or two, I began to feel dizzy and disoriented again, and I staggered across the hall to our bedroom to lie down. Within seconds of reaching the bed I realized it was happening again—I was really having a stroke! A more devastating stroke, affecting my whole body, not just one side, even more crippling than before.

All the previous symptoms returned and it felt like I was melting into the middle of a puddle of mud. I could feel myself losing consciousness and began to cry a bit, realizing this was probably the end of my life. I thought I was going to die and Monica and Willow would return home to find me dead. I thought, *How horrible for them.* I thought, *But I don't want to die!*

At that darkest moment, I heard the back door open and Monica's voice in a scolding tone to Willow. With what I thought was going to be my last breath, I called, "Mama," as I couldn't pronounce "Monica." Willow heard it and raced upstairs, Monica calling in hot pursuit, wondering where I was and what was going on.

I later found out that just a couple hundred metres from the house on their walk, Willow spun around, started to back out of her harness, and almost dragged Monica back home. They usually went for lengthy walks and Monica was in no mood or condition to fight with her, so she was going to put her back in the house and continue alone. It seemed like Willow knew I was in trouble, and this may explain her being all over me that morning. We've all heard the stories about the bond with pets and their ability to sense physical and emotional changes.

Monica called a second ambulance about 9:30 a.m. I can vaguely recall her talking with the 911 operator on the downstairs phone, describing the situation—what seemed to be another stroke. Our local ambulance had been dispatched to another scene since it was here earlier, so now we'd have to wait for one to come from the Stanley station, about forty kilometres away. I don't recall how long it took. I was still somewhat conscious when they arrived, but very helpless, just a blob.

This time it was a male and a female paramedic. They began to examine me on the bed, quickly assessed the situation, and saw that I needed to be transported to the emergency room of the Dr. Everett Chalmers Hospital in Fredericton immediately.

We lived in a 147-year-old church manse with steep, narrow stairs that can't accommodate a gurney, but luckily they had on board a stair-climbing chair/bed that they were able to strap me into and get me down the stairs and into the ambulance.

As the male paramedic drove as fast as safely possible, the female paramedic was talking to me the whole time in the back, trying to reassure me, telling me to not give up, to fight like hell.

She said her name was Niki. She was so kind and compassionate. I could tell she was experienced, and that gave me some needed comfort as we bounced along our way. With every corner and bump I was becoming more nauseous, and I even had to use a barf bag— that was a first. But they got me to the hospital, still alive, still having a stroke, and still very scared. I was so thankful for their help, but what now?

The paramedics wheeled me into the DECH emergency room shortly before 11:00 a.m. and immediately things swung into action. There were people constantly around my bed, either hooking things up to me or asking me or my wife questions. One was a former student I knew, named Victoria, now an ER nurse ready to deal with my situation. For the next three hours at least, it seemed like chaos. My right side would go limp, and I couldn't move my arms or legs or even talk; then I'd sit up and talk normally and be able to move all my limbs. Then suddenly my left side would drop out and do the same for a few more minutes, and then I'd sit up again feeling normal. I was vomiting or dry heaving each time one side or the other dropped out, and I was having massive leg cramps on my right calf and hamstring. The pain was intense and so was the sweat.

It seemed to me and everyone else that I was having a stroke, but my symptoms were atypical and no one could figure out why I was having a series of strokes on both sides of my brain. The looks of confusion on everyone who came in to help, the repeated questions we'd already answered, made it obvious to me they still hadn't figured me out and may not be able to do so. I could see Monica's frustration and concern growing, especially when they asked numerous times if I was on drugs. It was understandable they'd ask once, but over and over? I wasn't holding back anything, and it was getting on our nerves.

About three hours into the ER, the attending doctor asked a neurologist who was there treating another patient to take a look at me. The neurologist introduced herself as Dr. Bouma and began examining me, doing strength tests, and looking into my eyes with a light. I was still going in and out, I was losing muscle control alternating from side to side, and I vomited once again. After seeing something in my eye exam, she pulled my wife aside, and I heard her say she thought she knew what was happening to me.

She explained she would have to give me a clot-busting drug (tPA), which Victoria administered. After a CT scan, she said, they would send me to Saint John Regional Hospital (SJRH), an hour away, where they would try a fairly new procedure to remove the clots she suspected were lodged in my brain. Dr. Bouma made it clear that all this may kill me, but that if we didn't at least try, the outcome would be catastrophic.

Monica was terrified and frustrated with the long time it took to diagnose the actual problem, but at least now we knew what was happening. I was fighting for my life and was at least happy someone had figured out the type of stroke—a series of strokes—I was having. Monica and I agreed some hope was better than none, and even with the extremely high mortality rate, we had to roll the dice. I was immediately whisked off for that CT scan to confirm what Dr. Bouma suspected, and preparations began for my transport for hopefully a lifesaving procedure.

I knew the orderly who took me from the ER to the radiology department for that CT scan, too; she was another former student from the rural public school where I used to work. I was friends with her mom and had played softball with her dad. I could tell she was concerned for me, as was the radiologist giving the scan—the daughter of a good friend. I felt bad they were distressed about my situation. They felt my pain as I felt theirs.

Having never had a CT scan or MRI, it was so foreign to me—bizarre, almost, as I hadn't been in a hospital for much more than stitches or a cast for decades. Last time I spent a night in a hospital, I was almost three years old and had sunstroke on a family summer vacation in Prince Edward Island.

To further complicate matters, my ongoing leg spasms and massive beads of sweat were keeping me from lying still while they injected the dye and then performed the image scan. Another orderly had to stretch my foot and leg to try to keep me still. Just as I relaxed enough for them to try, the CT machine failed and they immediately ordered me into the other of their two machines.

Luckily, the second machine worked and I was able to lie still enough to get a proper scan. Dr. Bouma was in the screening booth looking at the scans as they were performed. They confirmed what she suspected. She had already called SJRH, and preparations were underway to have me transported there.

I was again surrounded by medical staff, Dr. Bouma, and Monica. Dr. Bouma told Monica I needed to be intubated and sent by ambulance immediately. I later learned that my type of strokes were in the brain-stem category, and the brain stem controls breathing, so Dr. Bouma wanted to make sure I could breathe during the transport and procedure. That way, as soon as I arrived at Saint John Regional Hospital, they could take me right to the medical theatre for the procedure with no delay.

Someone tried to force a tube down my throat and I tried to fight them off. Then someone said something about giving me a drug that would effectively paralyze me. Moments later I felt a needle, and within seconds I lay motionless, unable to fight, though I could hear them all doing their jobs, trying to save my life. It was terror to me. I was afraid if they put me to sleep I may never wake up.

When you're fighting for your life, it would seem to me the last thing you want to do is be unconscious, but I had no say. Before I went out, I saw some weird images, like the fins on a radiator moving forward and then to the right, and I remember thinking I may never see Monica's face again…and then there was nothing. I was out.

Chapter Two

The Early Days

On June 1, I woke, and no one was more surprised than me, although there seemed to be a few others in the room who shared my surprise. Within seconds, however, the joy of being alive was overwhelmed by the harsh reality of where I was, and the fact that I couldn't move anything from the neck down. I was more scared now than before if that was even possible. I could hear fine and comprehend in a somewhat foggy state, and I was alive, but now what? I don't recall anything between leaving ER in Fredericton and waking up in Saint John's intensive care unit.

I slowly began to realize who was around me. Some doctors and nurses mixed in with my family members. Monica and my sister-in-law, Joanne, were the first to see me. Monica asked Joanne to accompany her due to her nursing background; Monica wanted someone else in the room to remember things she would be told and may forget. She was still in shock and any help would be welcomed.

Eventually, my mother came in. She and Monica drove down the night before from Fredericton to be with me if I woke, though really they thought they would be identifying a corpse. Monica packed as many pillows as she could around the driver's seat to ease the back pain of a long drive. I was glad she could drive again, even if it was still painful, so they could be with me.

My youngest brother, Kevin, was also there. His wife, the former nurse Joanne, had had a debilitating stroke a few years earlier while in recovery from a brain tumour removal. She fought hard for years and has had a remarkable recovery. I helped take care of them both for some weeks as Kevin also had major health issues in the recent past, including a brain tumour of his own. Their faces told me all I needed to know—I was in serious shit.

In a few minutes, I could move my head a bit. I tried to talk but could feel a giant tube or two down my throat. My big Adam's apple has always bothered my throat, and the tubes were really stressing me. My wife could apparently read my eyes (and thoughts, like couples tend to do) and correctly conveyed to the attending nurse that she could tell I wanted the tubes out of my throat. She also warned the nurse that if I were to regain function in either arm, I would most likely pull the tubes out on my own. She knows me so well.

Just then a nurse popped her face in front of mine. She must have thought I was deaf or stupid, or maybe they're trained to talk like that when you're coming back from a near-death experience. She said slowly and loudly, "There will be a doctor by about ten or ten thirty to see you and hopefully remove the tubes."

She saw I understood, then pulled back from my sight, and I saw a big wall clock staring right back at me. It said 6:07 a.m.! *I have at least four hours to kill or be killed*, I thought. I started to stress again and tried to squirm. Monica reminded the nurse of what would likely happen if either arm began working again before that doctor arrived.

My right leg was still in spasms, adding to my pain and stress.

It was clear in this frantic scenario that I had to do something to calm myself down, to make it until that doctor could remove this damned tube, but what? I had a university degree with the equivalency of a double major, one in psychology, so surely I could think of something to keep me from losing my mind or my life, which I was fighting so hard for already.

I thought about seeing Joanne so courageously fight back from total paralysis and no speech, to walking with a cane, and then to speaking so clearly you'd never know she'd had a stroke.

I also thought back to when I worked with a young man who'd had a major brain injury from a car accident. He was in an induced coma for four months before beginning any rehab. He was using a wheelchair when I started working with him as his care attendant, and we would visit the Stan Cassidy Rehab Centre a couple of times a week for physio and speech pathology. Another couple of trips to a local gym through the week and me learning to stretch him properly all helped with his recovery. Within a year, he went from a wheelchair to a walker to a cane to walking on his own, although deficits still persisted. He regained his speech and was living life again at home, in the community, with family and friends.

I had a lot of inspiration to draw on. All these experiences were going to help me now that I was a patient, a survivor. I knew a little about neuroplasticity, the ability for the brain to change and adapt; to me it was mind over matter. I also knew that with strokes, the first six months of recovery are where you make your biggest gains. There was no time like the present to put all my knowledge, experience, and will into healing myself.

In the next couple of hours, my left side began to recover some feeling and function—I had tingling in my hand, arm, feet, and leg instead of complete numbness—so I knew I had some connection there, but nothing at all on my right side worked. I couldn't feel a thing, so I decided to stare at my right elbow, hoping I could make it move or at least try to make it move, until the doctor arrived to remove that damned tube. I remember mentally yelling and swearing at it to move. I had to start somewhere.

A STROKE OF LUCK

After a long time, three hours or more, it finally happened. My right elbow moved up a little, then back down. I was excited. Hope had made another appearance! My brother saw it move also and ran to tell a doctor. He returned with the doctor in charge of ICU, where I was placed squarely in front of the main desk for observation.

The doctor immediately asked if I could move it again, as perhaps it was just a muscle spasm. I couldn't talk yet but realized he was right, so I stared and concentrated hard on my elbow again, silently screaming at it. It only took about fifteen seconds and it moved again, up and then back down, same as before. It seemed to excite everyone in the room! I knew I had made a connection and the healing was beginning—or at least I hoped so.

The entire time, my right leg was in a massive cramp, and huge beads of sweat poured off me. A nurse wondered aloud why I was sweating so hard when my body temperature was cold. I remember screaming at her in my mind, *Lift the blanket!* I wanted her to see the leg muscles rippling in agony. She must have heard my telepathic plea, or maybe my wife read the situation again, because all of a sudden someone took off the sheet and it quickly became obvious what was happening. Again, the nurse stretched my leg to try and relieve the cramps, eventually succeeding for short periods.

After the team relieved my spasms and saw I was obviously improving a little, the ICU physician decided to finally remove the large tubes I had inhaled hours before. Monica told me later that when I was fighting them in the DECH emergency room earlier, it took three attempts to get them down properly, as my Adam's apple was giving them problems. She said a good-sized lad eventually just pulled my Adam's apple out of the way with one hand and put the tubes down my throat and sent me on my way.

When the time came to remove them, what a shock it was to the system. My mouth was so dry, my tongue had adhered to the rubber/plastic tubes, and it felt like they were tearing my stomach out, scratching my throat, and then ripping three strips off the underside of my tongue. I felt like a kid who'd stuck his tongue on a frozen pipe then pulled it off. It hurt like hell, but at least the tubes were finally out and my stress eased a bit.

I still couldn't talk. My left side was continuing to make progress. Though I was right-handed, Monica gave me a pen and paper so I could try to write with my left hand as the doctors talked to us about my chance of recovery or what I should expect for my future. I tried to write the name of a patient I had worked with in the past. It was sloppy, but Monica figured out what I was trying to say. I wanted them to know I had hope and would do all I could to get better. *Don't count me out yet.*

A STROKE OF LUCK

*

The next twenty-four hours consisted of hourly checks of blood pressure and a parade of doctors, nurses, and medical students through the ICU to witness the seeming success of the procedure that not only saved my life but would possibly allow me a better recovery than originally expected.

Dr. Bouma later explained to me that I'd had a vertebral artery dissection, a very rare stroke that she'd seen only once before, when she was doing her residency at McGill University in Montreal, Quebec. We all have two brain stem arteries, right and left. There is an unknown but substantial portion of people who have one side that didn't properly develop, meaning there is not enough blood flow to even sustain them if the other artery is not functioning properly. Most of these people live never knowing of the deficient brain stem artery because they can live with just one functioning artery. Unfortunately, I happen to be one of those people whose right brain stem artery doesn't work and I somehow tore my left, creating the chaos that nearly killed me.

The two walls of my torn artery began to separate, and the blood would sometimes flow in between them, perhaps explaining my stroke symptoms on both sides in the ambulance and in the ER. Eventually, it peeled the inner wall like wallpaper, creating a large flap that would block blood flow, and large clots formed behind it. Once enough mass and pressure had formed, the first clot pushed through and ended up in the centre pons region of my brain. Then another clot formed just behind the torn flap. Both clots had to be removed and the torn artery needed repair if I was to have any chance at all. The odds were stacked heavily against me; there was a very high mortality rate without treatment.

Dr. Brian Archer and Dr. Jake Swan were the interventional radiologists in SJRH who performed the procedure I needed. According to records, it was a couple of minutes after 6:00 p.m. when they started, and in under an hour they had gone in through my groin, up through the clot and torn artery, to the centre of my brain to remove a very large clot that had lodged there. After successfully removing both clots, they were now faced with what to do about the damaged artery.

Brilliantly, on their part, the doctors thought to try a heart stent, which has been used many times to open damaged arteries for heart patients. They had tried it with a stroke patient once before and had success, so why not try it with me? All options were on the table as, in my kind of stroke, any existing guidelines went out the window. Dr. Bouma had told Monica that we had to try—if we didn't do anything I would either die or be "locked in" from the eyes down, only able to blink for communication.

The heart stent worked, and imaging showed that perfect blood flow had returned to my brain. Now we all waited to see how I would respond.

A STROKE OF LUCK

Time is the biggest enemy with strokes. It is calculated that you lose two million neurons for every minute your brain is denied blood. My brain was completely denied blood for nine full hours, which equates to something like 32.4 years of lost brain mass, over a billion neurons gone. I was alive, but would I be kicking? Again, time would tell.

On my second day at SJRH, as I lay in front of the ICU desk, still scared and exhausted and willing the limbs and digits on my right side to move, the ICU doctor came to see me. I showed him I could now wiggle my thumb, index, and middle fingers on my right hand, and rock my right foot back and forth a little. I was trying to show him that I had made connections to my extremities. The right side of my face had drooped quite a bit and talking was very difficult—common with strokes—so showing him what I could do was my way of saying, "I'm not done yet!" He was stunned and said he'd never seen anyone make those connections that fast after such a long series of strokes. He seemed genuinely excited about it.

Monica and my mother had spent the night in a hotel and were back to visit me when the doctor made that remark. We all smiled and had hope. Today was better than yesterday, and no matter how little the progress seemed to be, it was everything to me.

I knew it would be extremely difficult for Monica and Mom to travel all the way to SJRH every day for who knows how long, especially as Monica was still recovering from her broken back. So,

I asked if there was a bed available for me at the DECH in Fredericton, which would be much closer to home for us all. I knew the staff wanted to keep me at SJRH for observation and perhaps for research purposes, but they said they would do what they could to accommodate my family and me. Within a day, I was told they had found a bed at the DECH and I would be transported by ambulance sometime soon. After one false start due to all ambulances being out on 911 calls, an ambulance and paramedics took me to Fredericton. I don't recall much of the trip, except for seeing the scenery go by out the back window and a nice paramedic originally from Saskatchewan keeping an eye on me and chatting the whole way. It took a little more than an hour and I was back in Fredericton. So now what?

I was admitted to 4NW, the acute stroke care unit of DECH, by a nurse named Christie, and then moved to a ward with three other gentlemen, who turned out to be ninety-two, ninety-five, and ninety-eight years old. In my confused, drug-induced state of mind and roller coaster of emotions, I saw it as the "goner" room. In my view, the doctors didn't think I was going to make it. The man next to me was hooked up to a bed alarm; he obviously had some form of dementia, talking gibberish and constantly trying to go to the bathroom even though he was hooked up to a catheter. I hadn't slept since they woke me at six o'clock the previous morning, and it didn't seem I would get any sleep soon, with all the noise and constant commotion around the room and the nursing station just outside our door.

The first nurse to come check on me, Juliana, made me feel welcome and tried to ease a bit of my obvious concern and confusion. She let me know Dr. Bouma would be in to see me shortly. Monica was there, too. Every time I saw her or my mom or thought of Willow and sometimes for no reason at all, I would burst into tears. I hated to have them see me this way and the stress it put them under.

Monica told me what was happening at home, that there were dozens of phone calls on our answering machine, people hearing rumours of what had happened, reassuring me that Willow was being taken care of, and letting me know the boys in our band wanted to come see me as soon as possible. I could talk a little by now, and I let her know to turn no one away who wanted to visit. It wasn't like I'd be sleeping anytime soon, and I certainly wasn't going anywhere.

Dr. Bouma arrived to examine me and talk about more CT scans and a possible MRI. It was nice to see her familiar face, even though we had just met a couple of days earlier. She'd saved me, in my mind, and I wanted to thank her for it. She downplayed her role, but when I later learned of how rare my stroke was, I was thankful she happened to be in the emergency room that day. I also learned from one of the long-serving nurses of the acute care unit that they knew my case was a big deal before I arrived, as it was the first time they could recall seeing a neurologist on the floor before the patient. She's an angel of mercy to me and I'm so lucky to have her on my healthcare team.

After she left, I just tried to take in my new surroundings, learn the new faces, and figure out how in the hell I was going to sleep. Friends started popping in on their way home from work or after they had their supper. It was so nice to see each and every one of them, in spite of my condition. I could see their concern and confusion as they entered. Maybe they were in shock, like my family. Their visits made me feel better, and hopefully they got some reassurance too.

Once visiting hours were over, family and friends of each patient in the ward had to leave. Night shift was underway, and the fun had only just begun in our room. Throughout the night, numerous alarms went off, nurses would enter and leave, and one patient had to be escorted to the bathroom often. Sleep was impossible for me, especially being right beside the bathroom. Also, I was still a bit afraid to sleep, fearing I may not wake up again.

So on through another long night and into the next day, not a wink of shuteye, only able to lie there, thinking and worrying, wondering what was next.

*

A STROKE OF LUCK

Day shift was in full gear, so it was another day for me of visits from nurses, doctors, and other medical staff, and it was Saturday, so more family and friends were able to come see me too. It helped the time pass and greatly distracted me from the physical and existential agony I was in, although it was all a blur.

At one point Charles Wilby, the drummer in my current band, The UnHeard, stopped by to see for himself how I was doing. Monica had tracked Charles down at his place to tell him how and where I was so he could share with our other band brothers, lead guitarist Vaughan Evans and bass player Bob Fitzgerald. They all stopped in that weekend. I was so happy they visited, but I cried every time I saw one of them. Everything seemed to bring a tear, which I was told is a common symptom of strokes; understandable, with such a shock to your brain.

As Charles sat on my bed, I asked if he had a cell phone with a camera. He said he did, so I asked him to take a photo of us and get it out on social media so people would at least know I was alive. Monica was going home and trying to politely answer fifty or sixty messages from concerned friends each night. It was my hope our photo would ease the burden for her so she could get some rest. She had been through so many traumas lately, I just had to do something to ease her stress. So out on the web the photo went, and after it was time to say goodnight again to family and friends, another sleepless night awaited me.

It was a repeat performance of alarms, entrances and exits by medical staff, assisted bathroom visits, lights on, lights off, my blood pressure cuff doing readings automatically every hour, and it all left me awake for a fourth straight day.

When I lived in Western Canada, I once stayed awake for four days, travelling to four different cities. I went from Vancouver to Kelowna by bus, then picked up an old muscle car to be delivered in Edmonton—but not before a pit stop to see friends in Calgary. I was much younger then and stayed up so long by choice. I never was a good sleeper, especially after years of shift work, mostly night shifts. I could operate now on four or five hours a night, but this lack of sleep in the hospital was really getting to me. I knew it couldn't be good for my damaged brain and body.

Another day of constant visiting, mostly friends, sometimes up to five around my bed. The other patients had visitors, too but my bed seemed to be the loudest. I have a tremendous number of good friends, many whom are also very funny and know how to use humour to lighten even the darkest times. Laughter filled the room many times that day, so much so I worried we'd all be kicked out. The families of the other patients said they didn't mind and thought it was wonderful to hear the laughter, so on we roared.

Some of the guys from my old band, Blind Dog, came by as well. One was Al, lead guitarist and vocalist. We wrote and recorded songs together back in the nineties. He lived away and we hadn't seen each other for a few years, only talked on the phone about the upcoming reunion at the Harvest Jazz and Blues Festival.

I didn't want to cancel the show. We had helped put the festival on solid ground in its infancy, and people were excited to see us return. I told him we would have to find someone to do my rhythm guitar parts and vocals but that the show must go on. When a doctor came by, I asked if it was realistic for me to be at the show only fifteen weeks away. He said it was a "nice goal," but I could tell he thought it was extremely unlikely.

When Monica arrived, the first thing she said was how nice it was to arrive home last night to only one message, which was just a hang up. She was able to go straight to bed, cuddle with Willow, and get some much-needed rest. I was so glad for her, and it told me the photo Charles posted yesterday must have done the trick! I asked her to bring in my laptop next visit so I could see for myself what was going on in the rest of the world. I could only use my left hand and my eyes were a little blurry, but I had lots of time, so why not try?

The most memorable thing that day, besides having the catheter removed, which I'd rather forget, was that a woman came to my room. She said she was a physiotherapist who'd heard of my case and wanted to see me for herself. It turned out one of the nurses knew her. The physiotherapist was a friend of Dr. Bouma, and the nurse told me how surprised she was to see her; she worked in private practice and had never been there on a weekend before. "You must be a big deal," the nurse said.

The physio had heard how quickly I was recovering some feeling and function on my right side. Still bedridden, I didn't feel like any of it was quick, but as each day passed I could tell something extraordinary was going on. Each medical person who came to see me appeared impressed by one thing or another—mostly with me still being alive against all odds.

The physiotherapist decided it was time to get me on my feet and try using a basic walker. That sounded good to me! My bad back was killing me, my ass had been sticking to the bed, and the cramping in my legs was getting worse. I hoped any movement at all would be a relief.

She left and returned with a walker, and for the first time I sat up and dangled my legs over the side of the bed. My whole right side felt like dead weight. Then with the help of the physiotherapist and with a safety belt on me in case I started to fall, I slowly got to my feet with hands placed on the handles of the walker, my left gripping fairly tight, the right just limply in place. It felt so good to spread my hips, stretch my back, and feel the floor under my feet again!

With the physio's close supervision, I walked out of my room right across from the nursing station and turned left toward the little lobby, which was maybe thirty feet away. For those few moments,

I forgot about everything and just enjoyed being in motion again and feeling a little hope. Today was better than yesterday. My new reality was changing almost daily, albeit at a snail's pace.

It didn't take long to walk a short distance with the walker, and the physiotherapist said she was satisfied and we should return to my room. When we got to the door of the ward, I refused to go in, and while drooling profusely down the right corner of my mouth and slurring my speech, I told her I wanted to go to the end of the long hallway and back. It felt so good to move I didn't want to lie down again so soon. She protested, but I ignored her and walked past my room and continued down the hallway.

She quickly pulled up beside me, grasped my safety belt, and whispered in my ear in a somewhat displeased tone, "I have been doing this since 1995 and no one has ever fallen, so don't you dare fall in front of that nursing station." I laughed and promised her I wouldn't and that I felt I could complete the walk, which I did. Down the long hallway and all the way back to my room before my ever-present fatigue kicked up a notch and it was time to return to my bed. I was pleased with myself, as were the nurses on duty at the desk, who seemed amazed at my accomplishment.

By Sunday night, when all the visitors had left, I knew again I wasn't going to be able to sleep. Dozens of bed alarms going off in my ear each night prevented any hope, even with earplugs. I hadn't pressed the buzzer for help since the whole ordeal started. I had asked for nothing and answered any question asked, but damn—I needed somewhere I could sleep!

When the head nurse for night shift, Kelly, came in to check on me, I quietly told her how I had been awake for days and asked if she'd help me out to the couch in the lobby or put my bed in a hallway where I could get some sleep. I even asked if she wanted to be the one who told the doctors their special patient had passed away due to sleep deprivation. I was desperate and she could tell.

At about one o'clock in the morning, two nurses entered my room and told me I was being moved to a semi-private room that had just become available. It was currently unoccupied, and while another patient was due to show up at some point, at least for the rest of the night I would have a room to myself, some peace and quiet, and maybe, just maybe, get some sleep!

The nurses gathered my things, released the brakes of my bed, and wheeled me out across the floor and down the opposite hall to a clean, quiet room. I finally had a window to look out. A window onto the world I used to know, not this world of chaos, care, and compassion. It looked like a full moon in the middle of my window. It was beautiful.

I thanked the nurses big time and thought this was just the ticket, Sandman here I come. Just as I was nodding off, my right calf went into a massive cramp, turned almost sideways. The pain was unreal, the acid and adrenaline were pouring into my stomach, the sweat was soaking my sheets and johnny shirt. I had been using a tension wrap or the foot of the bed to keep my foot stretched to prevent such spasms. I tried the foot-of-the-bed technique, but no luck. With the move to a new room, I didn't know where my homemade stretching device was, so all I could do was lie there in excruciating pain. A nurse came in eventually and stretched my foot and leg out enough to release the cramp and found my tension wrap so I could try to prevent it from firing again. I could only lie there, waiting for the next spasm—and of course got next to no sleep again. The only night I would have a room to myself, and I still couldn't sleep.

Monica had brought me my laptop, so at least I could listen to the radio and see what was going on in the outside world via the internet. After fumbling around from my bed and trying not to fall out of it, I finally got everything plugged in and attached to fire up my computer. It took about half an hour to do it all, and I still could use only my left hand at this point, but at least I now had access to the rest of the world. Wow, was I in for a surprise!

The picture Charles had sent out of us in my bed the other day had about 350 people acknowledging and commenting on it. My own Facebook page and our band page were full of best wishes and get well soon messages. I could barely use my hands but between the mouse and my left hand I started to try to answer some of them. I have the best friends and our fans are awesome! Everyone was expressing genuine concern and well wishes. People were stepping up to help both Monica and me. Still recovering from her broken back, Monica was trying to keep our large lawn mown, but neighbours offered to take over. Friends dropped off food and provided DECH parking passes and gas cards, which were especially helpful knowing the cost of travelling back and forth to the hospital each day.

After another sleepless night, even though I was now alone in a quieter room, I met new nurses assigned to me due to the move. A witty, cheery, British one came in and introduced herself as Debby, then took my vitals and asked if I would like to get cleaned up today. I hadn't had a shower in a week, as I never did get one before having the second stroke at home and being whisked away in the ambulance. I thought it sounded like a great idea and a chance to get out of my room as well, to get my bearings.

Debby brought me something to drink and my prescribed pills, which I choked down. Then off she went to see if the shower room was available. The unit had thirty-seven beds and only two showers—one in a good-sized room, the other in a small cinder-block room still large enough to accommodate a walker or wheelchair.

The smaller room was available, so Debby held my safety belt as I used my walker to get to it. There was a bench I could sit on, where I could lay out my soap, shampoo and conditioner, toothbrush, razor, and whatever else I needed to clean up my act. She turned the water on and adjusted it for me and showed me the string to pull that would signal when I was finished so she could come take me back to my room. I thanked her, she left, and I just sat there for a few moments, letting the hot water run over me.

As I started to wash myself and my hair one-handed, I began to have severe pain in my abdomen, or maybe in my intestines. At first I thought it was just some gas trying to escape. After all, I hadn't eaten anything for days, only liquids and pills, and every night I got a needle in the left side of my stomach to prevent thrombosis, so I was bound to have an upset stomach, right?

I finished washing and decided to try shaving with my left hand. A big mistake. I cut myself and began to bleed profusely, not realizing the blood thinners I was taking were preventing the blood flowing from my chin from clotting. Now the pain in my innards became unbearable, and I doubled over on the bench, grimacing. The whole time the small room was filling with steam, making it harder to get a breath when I could, between throbs of crippling pain. I realized I was in trouble and couldn't get to the string to pull to signal I needed help. Between the pain and seeming lack of oxygen, I could feel myself going into faint mode, panic mode.

Just then I heard Debby's voice asking if I was okay. I was barely conscious and called for help. She sprang into action, turning off the water, grabbing me a towel, and trying to examine me to see what was wrong. As more fresh air filled the room I felt better, and eventually the pain in my bowels subsided enough that I could get out of there. Debby helped me dry off and get some sweatpants and slippers on, then escorted me back to my room. She recommended I refrain from shaving for a while. I laughed and agreed, and Monica did too.

I'd heard other people say that when you stay in a hospital, you check your dignity at the door. With this latest adventure behind me, I realized just how true it was.

Once back in my room, I settled in to see what the day would bring. There were more visits from doctors and another CT scan—one of four or five I had in the first week. Dr. Bouma mentioned doing a couple of MRIs, one to see how my brain and the stent in my brain stem artery were doing, and one to check my lower back to see if my severe leg cramping had anything to do with a possible compressed spine. She explained how MRIs are different from CT scans and why they were necessary, then off she went, probably to see other patients or maybe to set up my tests.

About then, another patient entered the room and was transferred into the other bed. The hospital had told me someone would be moving in, but I was really hoping I would have a second day to myself so I could possibly get some shuteye. I was now at five days of virtually no sleep.

A STROKE OF LUCK

The nurses made sure the new patient was comfortable and told him they were aware of his condition and needs. Just listening to them I could tell it was a serious situation. I introduced myself once he settled; might as well get to know my new roommate, as it looked like we would both be here awhile.

He said his name was David Skinner and told me he had cancer, diabetes, and a host of other ailments that sometimes got so bad he couldn't stay at home and would have to come for stays in the hospital. He and his wife, Coleen, had a house just outside Fredericton, and they had a son, Lyle, who worked in Ottawa for a senator. David was a very proud man, I could tell.

As I told him of my escapades over the previous week, he was clearly concerned for me and very interested in learning more. For the next couple of hours, we got to know each other better. I loved his stories of growing up in Cape Breton and of meeting his wife when they both worked for CBC. It turned out many of the stories and images burned into my mind from my past news and political-junkie days were taken by him; he was an award-winning cameraman. I loved his slow and deliberate way of drawing me into whatever he was describing.

I mentioned I could see the back of the CBC building from my bed, and it turned out we had mutual friends working there. It is a small world indeed.

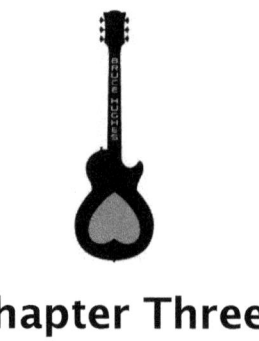

Chapter Three

Learning Self-Advocacy

David and I began each of the next few days listening to the local CBC radio show, critiquing the stories, guests, and sometimes the reporters. What we heard often prompted us to share another memory. We got to know each other really well, sharing laughs we needed—as did our loved ones.

When Coleen arrived, I got to know her as well, and came to realize what an incredible journey they had been on. At the age of forty, David had been diagnosed with cancer and given five years to live. The two of them had embarked on a wild ride, gaining every bit of knowledge they could, and had spent years chasing experimental drug therapies and test trials throughout hospitals in North America. It paid off, as David was now sixty-three, and Coleen sounded more like a doctor or nurse than a former CBC employee. What a love story.

One thing I knew and they reinforced is that you have to be your own advocate. It got me thinking about the discussion I had earlier with Dr. Bouma about the upcoming MRIs. Something about it just wasn't sitting right with me. Having no family doctor, I was assigned a hospitalist, Dr. Franks, a fine young local man who was easy to talk to and eager to help me any way he could. I asked him to get me some information on the stent in my brain stem artery so I could question Dr. Bouma on her next visit.

By the next day he'd printed off what info he could find, about not only my stent but also my type of stroke, which was much rarer than I realized. As I suspected, the stent was made of some type of magnetic alloy. An MRI machine, as Dr. Bouma had explained to me, is a large magnet, so I began to wonder if it was safe to do an MRI right now. Would it dislodge the stent—or even worse, just pop it out from the thin layers of skin covering the artery? It sounds crazy, but rare and crazy things were already happening to me.

When it was time for me to go for my MRI, Monica came with me, and we were filling out the questionnaire required. As I lay there, I peppered Dr. Bouma and another doctor about my concerns—which they seemingly did not share, as they told me they often did MRIs shortly after the placement of stents in hearts or hips. I asked if they'd considered that the heart has muscle mass and the hip has bone density to keep stents in place. Could they guarantee the MRI wouldn't dislodge the only thing keeping me alive? I half-jokingly remarked that I would hate to be an asterisk in a medical paper someday, advising doctors to wait six weeks for a heart stent placed in a brain stem artery to take root before doing an MRI.

As we continued to fill out the paperwork, the doctors realized I had asked a very good question. It was a rare circumstance, so they decided to consult with Dr. Archer and Dr. Swan, who had performed the thrombectomy and stent placement, and see what they thought. With just two questions remaining on the MRI admittance form and my anxiety growing, a staffer came through the door and said to not proceed with the MRI. Of the four doctors asked, only two thought we should go ahead.

The doctors decided to wait six weeks to make sure the stent was firmly rooted in the artery. I was relieved and happy to return to my room. Later, one of the doctors in favour of the MRI admitted they may have jumped the gun a bit, as they really wanted to see what was up as I was only the second person they knew with a stent in their brain stem artery.

David and Coleen's lesson of personal advocacy had paid off already.

I spent the rest of the day in our room, receiving visitors and sharing more stories with David. It was nice to talk to someone so interesting, and we laughed a lot. By the evening, it was time to try again to get some sleep. David was an old pro at sleeping in hospitals and seemed to fade easily. As usual, I just lay there, unable to shut my brain off. It seemed to be constantly racing to repair itself, afraid to waste a moment. And my leg cramps were always just on the verge of exploding, so I could never completely relax.

When my nightly stomach stab came, the nurse suggested maybe I take something to help me sleep. At this point I was ready to try anything, as I knew my body and mind were being further harmed, so I agreed to take a sleeping pill. Eventually I managed to nod off for a bit, but with the hourly bed checks and blood pressure machine taking my stats, it was only for short periods, minutes at a time.

Sometime in the night I had that feeling you get when someone is staring at you. I opened my eyes to see a woman, a nurse named Roxanne. I asked if she wanted some blood or was she if she was just checking on me. She apologized for startling me and said she had just come on the night shift and heard the other nurses talking about the "miracle man" who had survived a series of rare, major strokes and seemed to be making a remarkable recovery. She said she just had to come to my room and to see for herself if it was true. She worked with many stroke survivors, so seeing was believing. I thanked her, she left, and I managed to fall asleep again, although just for a few minutes.

When the regular routine of the morning came—getting my vitals checked, eating breakfast, and washing up—I couldn't get my head into the game; I was too groggy and disoriented from the sleep aid the night before. I just lay there like a lump until midafternoon. I was unable to do anything constructive and missed an opportunity to do some light physio work with the unit physiotherapist, Pam. I vowed to never take a sleeping pill again. My whole day was wasted in a fog.

I had yet another night of tossing and turning, short sleeps, and leg cramps, and then a new day dawned. After our morning routine, my friend Ed Hunter walked in. Ed was a cameraman at CBC I'd met years ago when I worked in radio. He's such a nice guy and great at his job. I always enjoyed chatting with him. We talked for a minute or two, and then I pulled back my curtain and asked him if he knew David. Of course he did; Ed moved over to talk with David for a while. It was a great chance reunion to witness. I smiled as the two of them got caught up on the latest at CBC and which camera gear they preferred.

Monica called the nursing station that morning and told them that when she came in today she would be bringing our dog, Willow! She had to get some paperwork done and then would be stopping by with her. Poor Willow hadn't seen me since I left in the ambulance. She had imprinted on me hard since we got her a year earlier through our vet. Both Monica and I have always loved animals, especially dogs. Willow played a part in saving me on the day of my series of strokes, but she didn't know it or what had become of me. I was beyond excited and began to bawl my eyes out thinking of her. I couldn't wait for her to visit. I knew I was in for a big boost to my spirits.

I could tell she was in the unit before I could see her. She is a very vocal dog, a cross between a border collie and an Australian shepherd, smart and hyper. I could hear staff and other patients commenting on how pretty she was and her barking back, maybe thanking them. She was definitely on a mission.

When Willow got to my room and saw me, Monica let go of the leash. Willow barked excitedly, ran to me, jumped on the bed, and began licking my face and making a soft, whining sound like she was crying. The floodgates opened in my eyes and I just hugged her and bawled. Monica joined us in a group hug and our tears of joy. My eyes still well up when I think about that moment.

After several minutes, Willow seemed to know I was okay and bounced over to my roommate David's bed to say hello, not even waiting for him to invite her up. She was like that, impatient and gregarious—like me, I guess.

Then she raced from the room and down the hall, announcing to others she was there or greeting them with a visit. She brought so much joy to the whole acute care unit that day. This was my best day yet—in spite of her being a bit naughty. We could all live with a little disobedience, given the circumstances.

*

During my seven days in 4NW, I got to learn more about what happened to me. Dr. Franks and Dr. Bouma were really good at answering my questions in layman's terms and getting me the information I requested. Everyone was so helpful, and everyone talked about how lucky I was or how amazing my recovery was. I still didn't totally understand what had happened, and especially not why, but I knew I was a big deal to them, especially the nurses who saw me every day.

Friends and family continued to visit, and my father even came from Cambridge-Narrows to see me. He looked nice in his best shirt and blazer. He recently had eye surgery to repair cataracts and didn't feel comfortable driving in the city, so my sister Susan brought him. He made a point to thank all the nurses and doctors that came to my room for taking care of me and saving my life.

I continued to get closer with David. He and his wife were two of the most amazing people I had ever met. What an incredible journey they had endured to extend his life and their love to the maximum limits. I had become more than a roommate in short order. According to Coleen, I provided a great stimulus to David, someone he could really open up to, share deep thoughts with. She also liked that I was an extra pair of eyes in the room to keep him out of trouble, especially when it came to his diabetes. His levels were all over the place, dangerously high and low, so both of them were meticulous with their notetaking; I did what I could to fill in the blanks when she couldn't be there to monitor dosages, timing, levels, etc. A buddy system had formed. We trusted each other.

One sunny day that week, I got to go outside. Each floor at the hospital has a patio for patients. This day my friends Dave and Brent came by, and my nurse arranged to get my food brought to me at a patio table. It was so nice to feel the sun and get some fresh air.

During our lunch, Dr. Bouma arrived to tell me she would like to do some more tests, to try to figure out why I was getting these leg cramps. I told her I would be up for anything that could help. Later that week, Dr. Bouma returned to take me to the lab for the testing on my leg. I was taken in a wheelchair to her office and lab and then to an examination room with a table to lie on. I got on the table, and she went to get her colleague who would hook me up and run the diagnostics.

The test involved Dr. Bouma sticking a needle-type probe into the centre of certain nerves in specific muscles. I was amazed at how precise they could be and how much it hurt when they would hit the nerve dead on. I was afraid my foot was going to spasm and kick one of them!

I peppered them with questions about what was going on with each exploration of the probe. There was an audio frequency assigned to the nerve, making it sound like a misfiring Harley Davidson motorcycle when the nerve was "on." It was silent when the nerve was "off."

Each probe, time after time, I would hear one or both of them say something like, "This just isn't right," or, "That shouldn't be happening." Was something wrong with the equipment, or was I really a freak of nature? Neither could explain what was happening with the readings, and the test was deemed inconclusive, so we would indeed add a double MRI sometime later.

I returned to my room and told David of my adventure that day. It was one he had never experienced in all his hospital escapades. He was beginning to lean toward me being a freak of nature—sort of like him. We laughed a lot about that. Two freaks, surviving any way we could.

That afternoon a pharmacist named Jackie came in, pulled the curtain around us, and told me she had just looked at my chart. "Do you know how lucky you are?" she said.

I told her I really didn't but would love to. She said it was the talk of the unit, that it brought such hope and joy to the staff to see such a success story. I still didn't quite understand their point of view. David cracked another "freak" joke when she left, and we laughed together again. Dark times call for dark humour.

After visitors for the day had come and gone and it was just David and I talking, he told me that during one of his hospital stays, he had somehow gotten himself trapped under the table they swing over so you can eat in bed. He thought he dropped something and was reaching to the floor to pick it up; regardless of he got there, he was stuck under the table and stuck good. He was alone in the room, and he had no voice at the time due to surgery and didn't think it wise to just wait for someone to find him. But what to do?

He could see a pipe of some kind running low along a wall by the floor, perhaps a water or heating pipe. Luckily, David knew Morse Code and brilliantly began hammering out "H-E-L-P" with his knuckle on the pipe. Over and over he called, not really knowing how long he tapped…it wasn't like he was going anywhere! Eventually someone noticed the tapping, though they didn't know the word, and followed the sound to David's room and rescued him from his self-imposed prison.

I wish I had recorded David telling that story—I couldn't stop laughing. He told such wonderful tales.

By Thursday, our room sharing days were coming to an end. After testing, I was approved to go to 3NE, the stroke rehab unit of the hospital.

With that bit of news, I began to gather what I could reach. Monica and some friends were there to help pack my bags. I was on the move again, this time from a place I was just starting to be comfortable in and where I thoroughly enjoyed the company and the incredible staff I had come to know. Both David and I had such great nurses, I knew a piece of them would be leaving with me to the next steps of my recovery. I also knew I'd be back to see them and David as soon as I could.

Midafternoon, I was transported down one floor to the ward, a room for four in 3NE. The bed I got looked like something out of an old cabin, a plywood headboard and footboard tilting to the right by a few degrees. There was what I called a stripper pole to the left of the bed going up to the ceiling, where a panel was gone so the pole could attach to something solid. There was some kind of industrial blower up there as well, making a lot of noise when it turned on.

How in the hell would I ever sleep? How in the hell was this supposed to help my recovery? But hey, at least I got a window, right?

I was fit to be tied and needed to get out of there and vent. I had seen an open outdoor space when we came in, and we vacated my room quickly to it. Everybody agreed, especially Monica, that we needed to leave before we said too much.

Why the hell were they moving me from a fairly quiet, stable setting to one that sent my stress levels off the charts? I had only had maybe a dozen hours of broken sleep in the last nine days, and this was unacceptable to me as a patient and as a human being. My body and brain were screaming at me, and anger was taking over. The outside space was my only salvation and solitude.

As we sat there trying to calm me down, a nurse came out and asked if there was anything I needed. I told her I would like a shower sometime. My last attempt with Debby hadn't gone so well, but I thought Monica could assist me; I couldn't stand yet and was still a fall risk. So, there we sat, waiting for a shower—and sat. Something had been lost in translation.

Hours went by. Monica and my other visitors all had to go, so I sat alone for a while. I was calming down some and dusk had come. There was a pillow left in a chair across the courtyard, and I thought about trying to sleep out there. It would be better than the bed and room I had been assigned, I was sure of that.

About then, another musician friend of mine showed up for a visit. Doug was a good man, like his brother and father. Our mothers were close friends and went to church together, so I knew the whole family. Doug had some experience in my new world; his wife worked next door at the Stan Cassidy Rehab Centre, an intensive care unit for paraplegics and other patients. He wanted to see for himself how I was doing, prepared for the worst.

After he heard my Coles Notes version of the last nine days, he could see how wound up I was. It was almost dark now, and the head nurse for the unit's night shift came out and said I had to come in. I told her I wasn't going anywhere until I had a shower.

It was then that they realized there'd been a miscommunication earlier. The nurses hadn't realized Monica would assist me in the shower; they thought one of them had to, and they just didn't have time. But my wife had been there for hours, more than willing to help me.

We were not off to a good start in "rehab."

Then the nurse made a fatal mistake. She told me I had to shave—not for any medical reason, but because "We like our men to be clean shaven"—and that I had to be in bed by ten o'clock. I refused both, reminding her this wasn't a prison. Who the hell did she think she was, demanding I do anything? She not only pissed me off, but in my mind, she had insulted Monica, who wanted me to grow a goatee for safety; she was all too familiar with how I had cut myself trying to shave with my left hand. My blood pressure and stress rocketed back to the top at this whole interaction.

She left and Doug stayed a bit longer, trying to calm me down again. He thought maybe I had been too harsh. I assured him I had not. I'd had a stroke; I wasn't stupid. She had no business telling me how I should look. To this day, it was my only negative experience throughout my journey.

By now it was about ten thirty. Doug would have to leave soon, and I would eventually have to go to my room, get my meds, and try to hunker down for another long night. I asked Doug to do me one big favour before he left. Would he come to the shower area and supervise me so I could sit in one of their shower chairs and clean up before bed? I wanted to send one last message that I'd meant what I said. Thankfully, Doug said yes. I really put him on the spot, but he awkwardly sat talking to me while I finally had a full shower. It felt so good and did help to relieve some of my stress.

I went to my room about eleven o'clock, received my meds, put in my earplugs, and waited for my eyes to close. No such luck. Even with the earplugs, the blower in the ceiling was probably still registering forty decibels of industrial white noise. It might as well have been screaming in my ear all night. Dawn was approaching and I was waiting for shift change. I wasn't going to stay much longer. Enough was enough. It was now Friday morning and I had a plan.

My roommate across from me woke and we made quiet introductions. His name was Henri, a leg amputee due to diabetes. I watched as he sat up and got in his wheelchair, gathered his bathroom gear, and headed out. When he came back we started talking. This was his second stay at the rehab unit. This time he was healed enough to get a new leg from the knee down and spend a few weeks in physiotherapy adjusting to it. He was thrilled he would be able to walk again. I was happy for him, too. He had such a positive attitude, I liked him immediately.

We went for breakfast together in the community dining hall. Many of the patients had breakfast and lunch together. Supper was optional; we could eat in our rooms or go out on a pass or have something brought in. Breakfast for me lately was liquid with yoghurt and a banana; hopefully the potassium would help with my leg spasms. Henri began to share his knowledge of the routines around here, who certain people were and why they were here. He knew most if not all of the staff. I'll never forget that first breakfast and how hard it was to try to eat with my left hand. I should have worn a bib like everyone else, especially after the second time my left hand missed my mouth, went past my ear, and poured the yoghurt down my shoulder. Coordination was another major deficit to deal with, especially learning to do everything again with my weak side.

After eating, I was taken back to my bed in the ward. I was told a physiotherapist would be by to assess me and discuss a plan going forward. I was in no mood for any of it. I was barely able to function at all, let alone think about starting rehab. How did they expect me to do much of anything? Was "Miracle Man" expected to be just that?

Within minutes a bubbly, smiling young woman approached me and told me her name was Maureen. Biggest, friendliest grin you could ever see. I could tell she loved doing her job and was serious about it. I let her finish her introduction and some small talk, and that was it. I went off on her, telling her I didn't care who she was or what she did. I told her I wasn't any good to anyone, including myself, unless I got some kind of rest. Why did they move me from my fairly quiet room upstairs where there was a chance of sleep to this hellhole of a room with a busted bed and loud noises coming from the ceiling above my head? How was this in the best interest of my health? I must have looked and sounded like a raving lunatic—perhaps I was.

Throughout it all, Maureen sat there with that big grin, taking all my desperate frustration without showing how hurtful I was being. It was the darkest day for me, and I've regretted it ever since. She didn't deserve it; she just happened to be in the wrong place at the wrong time. I even remember saying if something wasn't done I would check myself out and go home because at least I could sleep there.

Maureen left, realizing she was not going to get any cooperation from me today. I quickly began to put my plan into action. With the phone beside my bed, I called my mother, and without saying too much, asked if it would be possible for me to stay at her place this weekend. I knew I couldn't go home, where the bathroom was thirteen steps upstairs and Monica could barely take care of herself and Willow, let alone me. Mom said of course, so when Monica arrived that morning I told her something had to give or I was leaving.

By lunch hour, one of the nurses approached me and asked if there was anywhere I could go for the weekend, as they allow weekend passes, if approved, and there were no therapeutic services on weekends. I could get a pass as long as someone was there to watch me around the clock and I promised to return by Monday morning to begin rehab. Perfect! I could get out of there and still stay in the rehab program. It turned out better than I had imagined.

Both Monica and I felt our stress levels reduce immediately. Now we had to pack to leave for the weekend at Mom's.

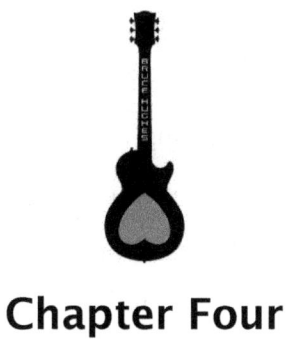

Chapter Four

Making Progress

Arriving at Mom's was the next best thing to being home. I was familiar with the house. Mom was a great cook, and I envisioned crawling into bed in the room at the end of the hall and sleeping the whole weekend.

We got all my stuff into the house, including my walker, which was a tight fit getting around in the kitchen or down the hallway. Mom had some homemade soup and rolls ready and we sat to eat. It was so good, so familiar, so comforting. For the first time in ten days I could almost relax, from exhaustion if nothing else.

As soon as I finished I went to the bathroom, a really tight squeeze in a small space for me and the walker. It was hard to believe this little bathroom, our only one, served all seven of us growing up. One sink, one toilet, one tub.

While sitting on the flush I looked at the bathtub and began to wonder how I was going to get in it, bathe, and get out on my own with only my left side working. Luckily, Mom had already installed a handrail, so I decided I would try a dry run later before attempting to sit for a bath. A challenge in my new reality I hadn't considered.

I thrashed my way out of the bathroom, bouncing myself and my walker off the door and walls until I got to the kitchen, where Monica and Mom were still at the table, talking. I was exhausted and said I'd like to go lie down. I assumed I would be in the little bedroom at the end of the hallway, but Mom had decided I should have her room with a much bigger bed and room to manoeuvre.

I knew she meant well, but that's not what I wanted. I wanted to be left alone to sleep as much as I could, which probably wasn't going to happen if I stayed in her room.

Too tired to argue, I dragged my butt, bags, and walker into her room and fell on the bed. It did feel good to sprawl on the queen-sized bed instead of the single at the hospital. Full-sized pillows, too. Mom and Monica asked if I needed anything else, and I didn't, so Monica was off to check on Willow and do some errands. Mom shut the door, and finally—silence. In a matter of minutes I could feel myself slipping away into dreamland. The elusive, much-needed sleep I craved was now going to be a reality…or so I thought.

Suddenly, I was rattled back to reality with a ringing telephone to the right side of my head. It was like a fire alarm had gone off; every nerve in my body was firing at once. While Mom had taken her portable phone from the room, she had left the charging stand on the night table by my head, meaning every time someone called—and she got a lot of calls—it rang in my ear.

To make matters worse, Mom usually put her phone on speaker so she could walk around and talk to the caller, the speaker always at full volume. The call that had just jolted me was from one of her many church friends, also the mother of friends with whom I grew up. The first thing Mom said was, "You'll never guess who is at my house." From there she filled her friend in on how I came to be staying at her place for the weekend and updating her on my health situation, like any mother would.

Every time I dozed off, the phone station beside me would ring, Mom would talk to the caller on speaker, often repeating the same story for each one. Not much chance of napping.

At night, I never slept more than two hours at a time between the always-present leg spasms or one of us having to pee in the middle of the night. I was still banging into the walls and having a hard time getting in and out of the small bathroom with my walker, so I started to leave it by my bed and grasp the door jambs to make a quieter entrance and exit.

By Saturday afternoon I figured if I couldn't nap I might as well try that dry run to get in and out of the bathtub without falling or drowning. I put the lid down on the flush and sat there thinking for a minute or two, envisioning how I would go about the task safely. After I ran the plan through my mind a couple times, I needed to test it. So, step by step I got in, went through the motions, and then got out, which was much harder than getting in. This without water and soap in the equation yet! I was successful in carrying out my plan, but I was exhausted.

I was always fatigued, and it took very little to play me out entirely. It made me think about how difficult the days ahead would be but thinking too much can defeat you if you let it. My motto was, "Deal with the present and hope for a future."

Saturday and Sunday were repeats of Friday, with daytime full of phone calls or visitors to the house. Mom is lucky, like me; she has great friends, full of care and compassion. They all wanted to wish me well, and some of them brought baking they knew I liked. The nights were similar as well, my sleep interrupted every hour and a half or two hours, whether by cramps or bathroom breaks. I only got about eight hours of sleep the whole weekend, but it was still more than I'd been getting at the hospital—I had only gotten ten or twelve hours of sleep in the entire nine days before I went to Mom's place. So, I didn't exactly feel rested at the end of the weekend, but at least I was beginning to feel some sanity return.

Monday morning came and it was time for the real deal—an unassisted bath. I gave myself two hours until we had to leave to go back to the hospital, knowing things never seem to go quite as planned. As the tub filled I brushed my teeth, shaved my cheeks with the new electric razor Monica had bought for me, and then slowly, carefully, crawled into the tub, all with only my left hand and leg to use.

When I finally sat down and began to relax a bit, it felt so good. I just wanted to soak in that tub forever! Eventually I began to wash myself and my hair. When I was finished, I pulled the drain and my attempt to escape began. The tub was a bit slippery, so it took me longer to get out than in, but I did it and sat on the flush again, exhausted from the effort but proud I had pulled it off. Independence was the goal of rehab, and in my mind, this was a major step.

I went to Mom's room, where I had laid out my clothes before I went to bathe. From my experience working with people with disabilities, I knew the difficulties of getting dressed, and I wanted to be prepared as much as possible. I got my underwear and socks on, though with some difficulty. Next were my pants. I had always put them on left leg first, just by habit. So, I sat on the bed, put my left leg in, then lay back and spent close to twenty minutes rolling around, trying to get my right leg in and my pants pulled up. Attempt after attempt ended in failure, and I was getting increasingly frustrated, but I was determined I would succeed. Finally, it all lined up and I got my leg through. Big effort for such a small success.

By the time I was fully dressed, shoes and all, I was so exhausted from wrestling myself that I was ready to go back to bed, not to the hospital to start rehab! Mom and my brother Kevin were there to see me and Monica off. I told them how worn out I was and described the battle to put my pants on.

Kevin laughed and said, "Bruce, you know better than that. The rule is always put our affected side on first." He was right, and as a care worker I knew that, but as a patient I had forgotten. Lesson learned; the next time I had a bath and got dressed, I shaved twenty minutes off my prep time from that tip alone! I also shaved some fatigue off too.

Now it was time to return to 3NE and see what the future would hold.

*

It was difficult to return, I must admit. Going back meant sharing a noisy, busy room and eating food that was just tolerable. I checked in at the nursing station and went to my bed to wait for their breakfast hour to end and the therapy sessions to begin at ten. I wasn't as refreshed as I wanted to be, but at least my head was clearer. Go time.

In my case the stroke rehab team (which consisted of the head of rehab, Dr. Bosse, Lisa the 3NE nurse manager, and many different therapists) determined that I would need lots of physio and occupational therapy, as well as speech pathology. As the day went on I met with the assigned staff, starting with Maureen, whom I had met and unfortunately exploded at on Friday. I was embarrassed by my behaviour and apologized. She treated it like no big deal. "We're here now, so let's move forward." Sage advice from such a sweet person. Maureen did some assessments so she could create a plan to proceed. We would work out together five days a week. I couldn't wait to get started.

Next, I met with Amanda, an occupational therapist who explained her role and assessed what I could and couldn't do with my right hand and arm and asked what my goals were. We had a pleasant, honest chat about what I should expect and how we could get there. She also did some assessments and said she would get back to me with a plan and schedule. I looked forward to working with her too, relearning what I used to do, or at least trying to. My fine motor skills depended on it. If they didn't return, I would never be able to play guitar again.

Up until this point, I hadn't thought about playing again—only that I didn't want to cancel our planned reunion. Once I started gaining some feeling in my right side again, I began to think there may be a chance to actually make music with my guitar again.

Lastly, I met with Sarah from the speech and language department, another kind, intelligent woman who talked to me about swallowing issues and what it was going to take to get the right side of my face to stop drooping and drooling so I could speak properly again.

My speech was returning very slowly. I had a few words but I was slurring a lot, very monotone, and had a hard time finding the words or pronouncing them properly. It was super frustrating and mentally draining trying to concentrate so hard. I would try to talk to anyone who came in my room for practice, hoping to speed up my recovery. I had watched my sister-in-law recover her speech from a stroke, so I knew how hard I was going to have to work at it.

On top of these three individual sessions, there were a couple of group therapy sessions. One involved hand and arm mobility and strengthening, while the other was circuit training. Each day there were four stations with various exercises and tasks, and we worked in small groups of four to six patients, with one or two staff.

In no time, my daily workouts began. The schedule was only five hours a day, but at first fatigue prevented any more. I jumped in with both feet—well, with one, anyway, and I dragged the other one along. It felt good, every session of all types of therapy, some harder than others.

I was getting to know some of the other patients better, especially in my group sessions or at mealtime. We always had fun at group sessions, joking with our instructors, Colleen and Joanne, or laughing with the other patients. We were mindful to encourage each other, too. I was shocked at first at how a one-pound weight felt like a hundred pounds in my affected hand, but with each passing day I could feel my hand and arm gaining mobility and strength.

One of the patients who sometimes participated in this class would often say inappropriate things to women. Most staff would just chalk it up to the stroke or his condition, but I wasn't buying it, and on more than one occasion I'd remind him that "harass" is one word, not two, to the quiet delight of both patients and staff in the room, patient and employee. It usually ended there.

Circuit class involved a variety of tasks, some for exercise and some for fun, riding a stationary bike or playing games, all in an effort to retrain the muscles and the brain to function like before. There were specific exercises for each muscle group, and there were some I couldn't do yet.

Dr. Bouma often came by to check on me and always said something about my progress, often adding, "We got lucky with you." One afternoon I showed her that my ring and baby finger on my right hand were still not working; it had been three weeks already and it frustrated me to no end. The other three fingers were working a little bit but were still numb and tingling. She said there may be long-term deficits in my abilities and that those fingers may never function fully again. Whether she meant to or not, she motivated me even more.

Given I wasn't sleeping much anyway, I spent that night pinning my thumb, index, and middle finger down on the table tray and willed the two that wouldn't work to move, like I did to my elbow after being awakened in the Saint John hospital.

By morning I was able to wiggle them a bit, and now they were tingling like the rest of my hand. I'd made another connection. It also gave me hope I'd be able play my guitar again.

The next day I saw Dr. Bouma in the rehab unit and I couldn't resist going over and showing her my movement. Her smile said it all—she was so proud and happy for me, and it made me feel good to see her excited for my improvement.

*

So now I had a plan, a schedule, and a routine. I knew it wouldn't be easy, but I wasn't afraid of hard work. I was only afraid that I wouldn't succeed, that I would never be independent, and especially that I would never be able to play my guitar again.

Would I possibly have to cancel the Blind Dog reunion show in September at the 2017 HJBF? And what about the band I was in now, The UnHeard? I had only met the guys I was playing with in the last two or three years, and we had a good thing going. We were playing some great music and got along really well. We already had some gigs lined up for that summer. I didn't want them to cancel.

With all the uncertainty, my brain was working overtime, trying to juggle everything in here and in the outside world.

Vaughan, our lead guitarist, stopped by to see me often on his way home from work. His mom was a retired nurse and warned him what to expect when he first came to see me in 4NW. Like the other bandmates, Charles and Bob, he anticipated the worst but was pleasantly surprised how well I was doing so shortly after the trauma I had endured. Still, no one thought I'd be playing guitar anytime soon. We had been trying out a third guitarist that spring, Dan, so I figured he could do my parts and the band could carry on for now—a relief to me, as I didn't want them to suffer because of my illness. I could focus instead on trying to pull off the Blind Dog reunion show.

As I settled back into the rehab unit and my schedule, the days seem to be passing quickly, but the nights not so much. I could feel myself growing stronger and steadier every day. Staff no longer considered me a fall risk; I was getting around pretty well with mostly my left leg and walker, so I finally got what I had been waiting for since I was bedridden in 4NW: a pee pass, as I called it. I was finally allowed to go to the washroom by myself! That might seem a small thing to most people, but to me and the other patients, it was a huge step toward independence—and perhaps a little piece of dignity restored.

I've been an early riser my whole life, so I was able to get up and go shower on my own at 5:30 a.m., before the rush was on for those who needed help. After all, I'd done everything on my own last weekend at Mom's, even though I wasn't supposed to. I didn't take chances when staying in the hospital, as I didn't want to have a fall and cause endless paperwork for staff. I never did fall during my rehab, in-house, outpatient, or at home.

After I did a successful stair test with Maureen, my team let me know I could have a pass every weekend if I wanted. I would have jumped for joy if I could! Lying on my nine-foot couch watching TV and snuggling with Monica and Willow sounded like heaven to me. It made the weekdays and nights more bearable knowing there would be some reprieve on the weekend. Others weren't so lucky. It bothered me that some patients had nowhere to go or no one at home to take care of them.

But for me, there was even more good news on the horizon. A bed had opened up in a semi-private room right in front of the nurses' station. Sleep deprivation was still a great concern, so I welcomed the move, although I was sure to let Henri and my other ward-mates know that it was nothing personal. I suspect the staff just wanted to keep a closer eye on me, and rightfully so given the severity of my strokes…and my mischievous nature.

I moved in and met my new roomie. He said his name was Keith but his friends called him Art. Or was it the other way around?

I just called him Art. He had some type of stroke after an operation to remove half a kidney or something. Turned out, much to his and everyone's surprise, Art was the only patient younger than me, but he needed and wanted to be cared for much more than I did. He stayed there on weekends usually, so after some more small talk I told him I was on a weekend pass and would see him on Monday when I returned.

I packed what I needed for the weekend. Monica arrived to get me. I signed out at the nurse's desk, where they also dispensed my meds, and we were off. I couldn't wait to see Willow and eat Monica's cooking, now that I could eat some solid foods, though swallowing was and probably always will be an issue, not uncommon in stroke survivors.

I don't recall much about being home any of those weekends. I just know they went by too quickly. Nonetheless, returning to rehab each Monday became easier, and I actually welcomed it; as long as I had a bed in the rehab unit, I would get therapy five days a week. Once I was discharged I could only get a maximum of two days.

My physio sessions with Maureen were going really well. She appreciated my willingness to work hard, and she pushed me every day. I loved working with her, but I'm not so sure she felt the same at first. I was always talking, releasing nervous energy, but Maureen felt it was taking away from my focus. She was convinced my bad knees would buckle at any moment and I'd fall, that talking would distract me from staying upright.

One day in speech therapy, Sarah introduced me to her summer student, Cynthia, who would be working me hard to get not only my speech back but also my singing voice. I mentioned what my physiotherapist had said about me talking too much. Sarah laughed, knowing me well enough by now to realize how impossible that would be. Besides, she and Cynthia wanted me to talk and sing all the time; it was part of my therapy. I laughed and said I couldn't wait to share that with Maureen next session, which I did, much to her amusement.

*

So, the days proceeded—physio, occupational therapy, and speech therapy—with small but visible improvements each session. I was feeling better, too, but my right leg still wasn't working much, and neither were my right ring and baby fingers.

I also had my eyes and ears thoroughly tested while there, my eyes to make sure no clots had formed behind them. I was curious to see if I had done any damage to my hearing with thirty-five years of playing loud music. I was sure I had and welcomed the examination. But it turned out I was okay in both the eyes and ears. Monica laughed when I told her my hearing was excellent. She said she knew all along that my hearing was selective.

A STROKE OF LUCK

Early each morning I'd greet the night nurses and take a shower, then go back to my room for my first coffee of the day and listen to Fredericton's CBC morning radio show on my headphones until about seven o'clock. By then, Henri would come find me and we'd take the elevator down to the little volunteer-run coffee shop in the lobby. It was Henri's first cup of the day, my second. We'd fight about whose turn it was to pay. We both ended up with coffee cards as we became regulars.

As we'd sit there waiting for our nine o'clock breakfast to arrive in 3NE, we would greet every employee, patient, and visitor. We were right by the bank of elevators in the main floor lobby, and it took no time at all to realize that, between the two of us, we knew at least half the regular staff and patients who entered the hospital. It was like a small city and we were in the only coffee shop in town. It was a wonderful start to the day, connecting with the outside world again.

Every evening, an elderly woman in a wheelchair would appear outside my new room. I had seen her at mealtime and sometimes in one of our group sessions. She'd sit and watch TV, and sometimes a nurse would bring some coffee, tea, or toast, after which she would often doze off in her chair. It was always so quiet in the evenings after all the visitors went home, just what was needed for the unit to rest after long days, but it drove me nuts. I still wasn't sleeping much, so I decided to go out and introduce myself to her. Her name was Helen.

Helen came from the small border town of McAdam. She had worked in the bank there for forty-seven years and was here waiting for a nursing home bed to open, somewhere for her to live out her remaining days. She was a sweet woman with a great sense of humour, in spite of her weakened body and situation. Her only living family member, her brother, was one floor above us in some type of critical care. She visited when she could.

We would talk the evening away, laughing at each other's awful jokes or teasing each other. Sometimes I would go get us coffee and share some of the baked goods Monica made me on the weekends. Helen had a sweet tooth for sure! We always complained about how bad the coffee was, so I told her I'd bring in a jar of my favourite instant next week and she could help herself to it. It had to be better than the coffee in our unit.

Other patients began to appear at our evening sessions around the TV, coming out of their rooms and shells to share in the laughter and the coffee and the treats. There was Henri, Fred, Anita, Sam, and many others. Some evenings their family members would join us and we'd end up one happy bunch, taking up most of the lobby area with double-digit, standing-room-only crowds. Reality TV had a whole new meaning.

When the first jar of coffee was gone, we decided for fun we would start a toll to get past our evening TV mob, to replenish our stock. I called it the Coffee Mafia and Helen was the one, in charge of collecting the tolls. We even made a little sign and left it there overnight. Much to our surprise, some would throw change in when we weren't looking, and when we had enough we'd buy another jar of coffee for any patient to use. We were taking care of each other, sharing the load, the spirit, and the laughs.

There were evenings I thought someone would come tell us to calm down or that we were being too noisy, but it was the complete opposite. Lisa, the nurse manager of the rehab unit, thought our group was marvellous. Working in the stroke unit was hard but rewarding. The nurses saw people's worst days, some patients they could only comfort, not help, and there were some who didn't make it. The noise and laughter they heard each evening from us was music to their ears. It was hilarious to us patients, but it sustained us all, like group therapy should. Humour is great medicine.

One nice day in July, we had a late afternoon gathering with about fifteen patients and family caregivers out in the open space. It was a large patio with chairs and plants, and we were all gathered under a canopy for shade. Everyone was happier and more relaxed in the fresh air. Sometimes I'd throw a towel over my arm and act as their waiter, bringing them coffee and treats or water. We were having such a good time outside we thought it would be nice to have our supper out there, but we were told no because of such short notice. We begrudgingly went to the dining hall or our rooms as usual, but we hoped we'd be able to picnic someday.

I would often go out there on my own, to soak up some sun or just get away from the noise and bustle inside. Sometimes Cynthia would find me there and have me do some tongue-twisting exercises for my speech, or Amanda would bring me the latest device or game to test my fine motor skills.

Maureen's kids had sent me their personal mini net and basketball, and Megan, the physio assistant, set it up so we could shoot hoops. It was so sweet of the kids to do that as they knew I used to play basketball and they wanted me to do it again.

I liked being in that outdoor space, but it was ugly and dirty and certainly underutilized. A volunteer, Leslie, had put some potted flowers around and tended them, but that was all the effort going into the space. I'd pick up any garbage that had blown in or been left behind. There were bird-shit stains, and gravel that must have fallen from the roof above. The gravel impeded some people in wheelchairs, and a fall might mean embedding gravel in whatever part of your body hit the ground. I often threatened to bring in my shop vac and clean the place up myself. One day, I did just that.

Monica brought in the shop vac and a long extension cord. I decided rather than clean it all I would only do half so people could see how nasty it was. It was a 34°C day. My visiting friend Dave and fellow patient Sam were there. Neither thought this a good idea, but at least if I had another stroke we were just steps from the hospital doors. It was hard work, but I was determined, and I knew I'd be building strength and independence, too. Besides, the patients deserved to have some fresh air and sunshine in a space as inviting as possible. Everyone inside was busy, so why shouldn't I do it?

After two hours of work spread over three or four sessions broken up with shade and a water break, I'd cleaned up half the space. The difference wasn't as dramatic as I'd hoped. People were peeking out of office curtains, wondering what the hell I was doing. Others, I heard later, were concerned I'd have another stroke, or get heatstroke or sunstroke. The nurses knew I wouldn't listen to anyone, but I'm pretty sure RN Rebecca was watching just a few feet away the whole time, just in case.

As summer flew by, my physio, occupational therapy, and speech therapy were progressing well. I had upgraded from the static walker with two wheels and two legs to a four-wheeled walker, and I could move around quickly when going for coffee or to visit my friend David back on 4NW. Daily we would check on each other, taking turns visiting each other's unit, chatting and bantering as friends. I had the utmost respect for him, and a day didn't seem complete without a visit.

Chapter Five

Homeward Bound

As much as life was getting better for me, there was one thing I hadn't even started working on yet, and it was the thing I wanted to do more than anything else: play my guitar.

I had already set forth a plan for the Blind Dog reunion show, to hire one of our former band members, Craig, to play my parts. I hoped I could at least be there that night to support the boys, even if I couldn't play. I booked four rehearsals over the summer and paid for them myself; two of the guys would be travelling from away, so I thought that was the least I could do. Most Blind Dog reunion rehearsals and The UnHeard practices were on weekends, so with my weekend passes, I was able to attend. It felt good to be in public, listening to live music, but it was killing me not to get up and play.

I was missing that inexplicable euphoric feeling I get only when I am playing guitar.

One day, Amanda told me to bring my guitar in when I returned from the weekend and show her what I could do. I had picked it up when at home on weekends but barely had the strength to hang on to a pick, let alone the guitar. I had no rhythm at all and could barely move my hand back and forth in a strumming motion.

When I brought it to a session with Amanda the following Monday, I found that I couldn't even get my right shoulder over top of it without fatigue setting in immediately. I tried to strum with the back of my index finger and I couldn't coordinate my hands. The sounds coming from the guitar and my monotone voice trying to sing were awful.

Amanda had shown me early on an exercise that would test my coordination, involving tapping my feet together quickly. If I could master that, my coordination would be back. The first time I tried it, I was shocked at just how out of sync I was. To this day, I do this exercise to improve coordination, but at that time, I knew I was nowhere near ready to perform. It was the first time I felt a bit depressed. But all I could do was put it away and wait another week and try again. It was a huge disappointment, but I tried to see it only as a delay and not as a defeat.

Amanda, always the optimist, put her best spin on it. She didn't think it was so bad and thought we'd get there eventually. I really wanted to believe her, but in that moment I had my doubts. Early on she had given me a "grasp bag" of tools to work different motor skills alongside some real-life tasks. The bag of tricks, if you will, had a lot of items to strengthen my grasp, but nothing to simulate the back-and-forth motion of playing guitar. I thought of an egg shaker, but I couldn't have held one in my picking hand.

The next time Amanda worked with me, she passed me an ingenious little device she had made from two very small disposable pill cups with some dried rice in them, all held together with electrical tape. Not much to look at, but it fit perfectly between my thumb and index finger and stayed in place when I shook it. I could mimic the motion of playing, strumming up and down. Eventually I began to change the rhythm patterns, too. I couldn't thank her enough. Finally, I could see some light at the end of this dark tunnel.

The hands are often the last to return, having the finest motor skills of all. It takes three sets of muscles just to close and open a fist. With only a few weeks to the reunion show, it was looking less likely I'd be able to play the whole set, but this gave me hope that maybe I could improve enough to do at least a couple of songs. There were still some rehearsals to go, so a lot could happen between now and the show. It felt like my dreams had been delayed, not dashed.

By July, about a month after my series of strokes, I'd made improvements in all my sessions. I was walking, rarely using any kind of walker. Granted, I wasn't a pretty sight to see walking, my right leg dragging along. Maureen was doing the best she could with me, but at one point we sat down with a doctor and discussed what to do about my knees. Maureen said my legs were like a bad set of oars—my feet went one way, my knees the other, then they all went SNAP, and somehow I walked. She often walked with a hand hiding near the small of my back, ready to grab my safety belt if I went down. I couldn't blame her; my knees were so sloppy from my sporting days and I had fallen before my strokes. My options were braces, surgery, or just carrying on. I was glad we decided against surgery; I was just getting on my feet, and that would put me on my back in bed again. I would have to find a way forward instead. I had some neoprene wraps from my basketball days. They would do for now.

Cynthia continued to challenge and test me on my speaking and singing. She once gave me an exercise of sentences that had me tongue-tied in half an hour. No one ever had been able to silence this tongue—not my teachers, nor my parents—and she did it in thirty minutes! I begged her not to let anyone know her secret formula and we had a good chuckle over that and something about blackmail money for a poor student maybe. Both Monica and I liked her. She had a great sense of humour and an awesome ear for just the slightest difference in sound. I learned a great deal from her and still pull out those exercises every now and then.

With weekend passes and now sometimes nightly ones, I started to go to summer concerts and barbecues, to mow the lawn, to get out on the town with Charles, Vaughan, and Bob just to hang out and have a meal together, and once to watch them play at River Jam. I spent Canada Day with my friends John and Debbie at their place, where they had their annual summer bash with live music from some old friends. Sunday rehearsals for the Blind Dog reunion show were the icing on the cake.

One weekend at home I even got up the nerve to get a walking stick and try to get down the partial stairs to the river so Willow could go for a swim and a river walk. Now, that was an adventure—slowly sliding down the steep bank a couple of feet at a time, with the walking stick digging in on the downhill side, hoping I didn't lose balance and fall in the river or hit my head on shoreline rocks. I finally made it down and waded into the river.

Life was getting better, but I wanted more, so much more. I wanted my whole life back.

*

By the middle of July, I knew I might be discharged soon. My progress was remarkable, I was told; seeing the other stroke survivors around me, I finally realized it was true, and I was very thankful. You're supposed to be discharged when you are capable of taking care of yourself at home with minimal assistance. I was pretty much there, with the exception of driving, but some clinicians were happy to have me stay a while longer so they could do tests and exercises they never could do with other patients. I loved all the gadgets and games they tested on me and I was glad to give them some data for future reference.

I was trying to help around the unit, too. I would move chairs around at mealtime, pass out the bibs, make toast for patients smothered with Monica's homemade jams. Most evenings I was still making a round of coffees, usually with treats, for Helen and me and whoever was sitting with us.

Sam and I had become good friends. His wife, daughters, and grandchildren visited him often, and Monica and I spent a lot of time with them in the outdoor space or around the TV. I often visited with him in his room. He had some serious health issues and seemed content with just sitting around in the day, not wanting to participate in much. He would watch me, though, busting my ass to get better, amazed at how far I had come in such a short time. I was hoping I could inspire him to keep fighting, to never give up. Nancy and his daughters appreciated the efforts and often told me so.

One thing we had in common was our hatred of the fishcakes on the menu. We nearly started a riot one supper after twenty-three of twenty-four people threw out their fishcakes. We figured out they were fishcakes only because of the tartar sauce packages on our trays. These "fishcakes" looked and tasted like a combo of pocket lint and sawdust. The second time they appeared for supper, I was ready to find the person in charge of the kitchen and ask why the hell they were still on the menu. What a waste of money and food, I thought. Hardly anyone ate them.

Sam and I had such a good time hanging out, laughing, sharing our stories of yesteryear, usually with salty language. One day his daughter said, "I'm glad you two didn't meet in your youth, because I'm sure you both would have ended up in jail." Well, we had indeed become thick as thieves.

*

Some patients had come and gone in our rehab unit, but others had arrived before me and were still there when I left. Seeing your name on the discharge board was a big deal and meant you were leaving to embark on the next phase of recovery, or at least a home where you could go live in the real world. Some patients had gotten better; some had healed as much as they were going to and knew they needed assisted living now. I was determined to be discharged and resume the life I had or as close to it as I possibly could get.

Every Wednesday, the head of the rehab unit, Dr. Bosse, would have an afternoon conference with the staff to discuss the patients' progress. You didn't get on the discharge board without her approval, and not until they had done all they could do and you were well enough to go home. I checked the board every Thursday morning to see if my name was at the "Top of the Pops."

I was mentally ready to go home, even if not completely ready physically. I had been in hospital for nearly seven weeks. Whenever I was discharged, I would keep doing two days a week of therapy in the outpatient program. My right leg still wasn't working very well, but I dealt with it, keeping up with the exercises Maureen had shown me, the footboard stretch, and walking as much as I could when I was home on weekends.

I was beginning to take my guitar out more, still playing terribly and unable to hold a pick, but I knew it was the only way I was going to get better. There were rehearsals coming up for the reunion show with Blind Dog, and The UnHeard had a couple of gigs I wanted to go to as well. I thought I could maybe even get up and say a few words or sit in for a couple of tunes.

As I returned one Monday morning for what would be my last week at 3NE, I realized how close I had become to the staff. So many of them were pulling for me. My success was their success too. I could see them from my room whenever I was resting or sitting with Helen watching TV. Lisa, the nurse manager, was easy to talk to and well respected by the staff and patients. Her calmness and big smile were infectious. All of the nurses had become like family to me, the ones on 3NE and 4NW too, where I visited almost daily.

A nurse, Rebecca, asked me to meet her at the main desk at 3:30 p.m., shift change, that Monday. When I arrived, a few of the nurses were standing there, so I knew something was up. On behalf of the staff, Rebecca presented me with a tag made from a paper pie plate and a paper clip. It said:

Bruce Hughes

Honorary Staff

I'd been working hard to regain some control of my emotions, but I was so touched by this it was a challenge not to cry now. I finally managed to say, "Thank you, but I don't think this will get me through security!" I hugged as many of the nurses as I could. It means a great deal to me to this day. They all played a part in my success, and in their world I was an example of the reason they do what they do.

Hope is eternal. Compassion is priceless. Success breeds success. I can't say it better than that.

I eagerly awaited the weekly Wednesday conference to see if I was deemed ready for discharge from 3NE to start the next phase of my recovery as an outpatient.

After arm class and circuit training, Amanda, my occupational therapist, had me try lots of new gadgets and games, testing my strength, speed, and dexterity, recording improvements daily. Maureen continued to make me sweat each physiotherapy session, and I was gaining strength and mobility, but I could tell she still wasn't convinced my knees were going to hold up. I assured her I'd be fine. Cynthia was winding down her summer assignment and would bring me more tongue twisters and photocopies I could take home to work on my speech.

Every single one of them had done their very best to accommodate my every deficit and I had improved in every aspect. How could I ever thank them enough? Even if I didn't improve at all from here, I'd regained a quality of life I could live with, thanks to them.

Thursday morning arrived. I had my usual early shower and coffee, then went down to the hospital lobby to the coffee shop for a second cup. By now I was like a fixture, with staff and visitors saying hello or commenting on how well I looked or how far I had come in my recovery. I think we all need encouragement to deal with major life changes, especially such traumatic ones.

When I went back up the elevator for breakfast and rounded the corner to the nurses' station, there it was. I was at the Top of the Pops, the first name on the discharge board: *Room 45B—Bruce H—Friday July 21.* I felt pure joy, seeing my name on the board.

It was official: I was going home. A few of the nurses waited to see my reaction; they were as happy for me as I was. It was a moment to reflect on all the hard work by me and my rehab team to get to a point where I was going home, not to a special care home. There was still room to hope for a full recovery.

Amanda told me during the day's therapy session that she had recommended me to the director of therapeutic services, Patti, as a candidate for the volunteer position of Patient Experience Advisor (PEA). They had an opening, and my cognitive abilities didn't appear to be affected by my strokes (although some may disagree). The position would allow me to stay in touch with everyone and give back to those who had done so much for me. I told her I was honoured to be asked and that I would be interested in finding out more. After all, occupational therapy is about doing things again, participating in life again. It made me feel proud and useful.

I knew I only had one more day to say goodbye to all my hospital friends. I felt a little guilty about leaving them. I sat with Sam for breakfast. He was really happy for me, but I knew he would miss our chats and banter. I would, too. I loved hanging with Sam, and I wished I'd met him earlier in life. I promised him and all the other nurses and patients that I'd come visit.

After the morning therapy sessions were done, I had a little time before lunch, so I went up to share my good news with David in 4NW. He was thrilled for me and Monica. He knew how important it was to get home, having spent so much time away from it, both for CBC and in various hospitals throughout North America trying to stay alive.

I was elated and honoured to celebrate his sixty-fourth birthday with him in the hospital, even though we had wanted to do it at his home with Coleen. David's health had taken another turn for the worse and he was now waiting to hear about a possible transfer to a Quebec City hospital in a last-ditch effort to prolong his life. He was convinced he would beat the odds again, not to worry.

"We all have to go sometime" has more than one meaning; in my case, it was time to go home.

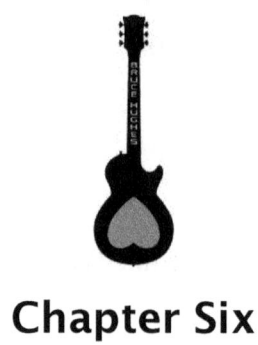

Chapter Six

Back to Music

D-Day. Discharge day. It had been an incredible fifty-one days since my stroke. There seemed to be a buzz in the air that morning, or maybe I had too much coffee. I'd packed most of my things the night before, though it would be mid to late afternoon before I could go.

As I said goodbye to the other patients, I felt torn between my happiness and a twinge of guilt for those who had been there longer than me or hadn't recovered as well. I would always tell them to never give up; it was mind over matter, and I was proof. Hope and inspiration were all I could offer, with a hug or a handshake. I know they were happy for me.

I took one last trip to see David and say goodbye to the many wonderful nurses and staff on 4NW who took good care of me as well. David was so pleased for me. He told me how much he'd enjoyed getting to know me. It was an honour and pleasure to become friends with him, truly one of the most interesting people I had ever met. I told him I'd stop in at least once a week to see him and Coleen and looked forward to finally meeting his son, Lyle, who was flying in soon for a visit. David was so proud of him.

After some emotional goodbyes, I went back down to 3NE. Monica arrived, we gathered my things, got the paperwork done and medications figured out, and off we went, in tears. I left a message on my writing board on my pillow for the nurses to read. One of my old friends, Dave, who would visit often, had started calling me Pedro when I grew the goatee, so my sign said, *Pedro Hughes is gone fishing.*

We had nothing planned for that weekend. I just wanted to lie around and see how I felt. A few friends and a former student stopped in on Saturday. Sunday consisted of eating and going into the field a few times with Willow and learning to throw a Frisbee again. My strength and accuracy were terrible, but Willow would go get it anyway. I could tell she really missed our time together. When I would go lie down with fatigue, often on my right side with a pillow between my knees, she would come up and curl into my stomach, then fall asleep. She wasn't letting me out of her sight now that I was home for good. It felt good to be snuggled again, for both of us.

My outpatient sessions were booked, I had new physiotherapists to work with, and I was lucky to continue my occupational therapy with Amanda.

Later in the week, my UnHeard bandmates, Vaughan, Bob, and Charles, had an evening gig at one of my favourite local spots to play, the outdoor Lawrence Amphitheatre at Nashwaaksis Commons. It had been booked before my strokes, so they were going to try a trio version of The UnHeard, with the plan for me to join them for two songs at some point in the ninety-minute set. I couldn't wait, even though I still couldn't play very well. At least I could sing a bit better.

A few songs into the set that night, they called me up to the stage. I hobbled up to a nice round of applause; there were a lot of friends in the crowd that evening. We decided earlier I would play acoustic guitar only and sing a Tom Petty cover tune and one I had written. After I got through the first number I turned to the band and readied to go into the second song, but we didn't.

Vaughan looked at me. "Are you going to start it?"

I replied truthfully, "I can't."

This struck us all as funny and we were laughing as Vaughan took over my part as well as his own and off we went, playing "End of Nowhere," which hopefully it was.

It felt so good to finally be back playing with them again, even if it was too brief and I was awful. It was another step on my road to recovery. I couldn't wait to get back with them full-time, but first I had to get ready for the Blind Dog reunion show, less than two months away.

We had one or two more rehearsals for the reunion, and my spirits were high after sitting in with The UnHeard. I began plunking around and seeing which songs I might be able to play rhythm on. Three quarters of our set that night would be original material Alan and I had written, some of it as long as twenty-five years ago. I still couldn't strum very quickly or hold a pick, so the simpler the better, I figured. I tried to find songs I could get through without too much embarrassment.

At the next rehearsal, I tried out a couple of songs and announced I would get up at the end of our set for the last three songs and sing lead vocal on "End of Nowhere," which I had written the music and most of the lyrics for with Alan. I wasn't sure it was possible, but I was going to keep working toward my goal of being on that HJBF stage again.

Summer was short for me. I really only had August to soak up some sun and see everyone. With limited energy, I had to make my ongoing therapy sessions at outpatients a priority. And because I needed a drive to go anywhere, I was home most of the time. People had to come visit me for the most part. It sure was nice to see anyone and everyone at barbecues, concerts, or just in the yard.

By September the Blind Dog reunion rehearsals were over, the songs were selected, and I could play the last three songs okay. It wasn't what I wanted, but much better than anyone would have guessed I could do three months ago.

There were radio and newspaper interviews set up to promote the show and to update folks on where I was in my recovery. Word had circulated that I was going to be at the reunion in some capacity. Our bass player, Dave Cunningham, and I did all of the interviews, and our other bandmates participated in some as well.

Dave has such a great sense of humour. It was a blast doing the media circuit with him. We had become really good friends over the years, even though we hadn't played together in a while and didn't see much of each other once he moved to town. Any time spent with Dave is a treasure to me. He's the type of guy who doesn't say much, but when he does, you listen. As a musician, I have more respect for him than anyone. Can he play!

For each interview, someone had to travel out and get me—an hour-long round trip—then drag my butt with them all day until Monica got off work, or they'd have to drive me home too. Dave handled one pickup and delivery; he was retiring and had time. For the rest of the week of interviews, my old high school friend Len Lynch became my chauffeur. He shut down his business for three days to get me where I needed to be until the reunion show was over.

He promised Monica he'd keep an eye on me, especially my fatigue levels.

We had a Blind Dog interview at 95.7 The Wolf, where I used work, with station manager Conrad Mead. It was always fun to be on air with Conrad, he himself a trumpet player. He and Dave had played many years together in the Downtown Blues Band, where Dave landed after Blind Dog disbanded. It was like Old Home Week, sitting in the studio for that on-air chat.

We also did a radio segment with my friend Roger Jean at CHSR, the University of New Brunswick (UNB) station, my alma mater. We talked and Roger played some of our old songs, which is always special. Roger liked both the old band, Blind Dog, and the current band, The UnHeard—he'd been at a couple of shows in the past year.

While on campus, we sat down after the radio interview with reporter Ryan Gaio of the student newspaper *The Brunswickan*. Ryan is an outstanding young writer. We had a blast with him and he captured the spirit of the occasion very well in his story about the reunion.

Next, we were off to a CBC radio interview. It's always fun to go there; I did many interviews in different capacities in my working life on radio. I got to know several staff, including a young woman, Lauren Bird, who I mentored in her senior year of high school on my old radio show. She was there at CBC that day, doing what she'd always dreamed of, journalism, and had just taken an offer to do some work at the BBC in London, England. I was very proud of her and happy she happened to be there when we were doing the interview. I went to high school with her parents, fine folks who, like Lauren, always thanked me for helping her get started and believing in her.

Again, Dave was funny as hell without even trying to be, making for a good three-way chat on air. My favourite part of the interview was Dave telling about his first visit to see me once I was transferred back to the hospital in Fredericton. Monica had called him and filled him in. Dave told Lauren about how worried he was, knowing strokes can be so debilitating. Then he continued, "I went into the hospital the next day, he's sitting there talking a mile a minute, waving one arm around, anyway, and now he's walking and talking, almost getting there." Cracked me right up!

As we left the building and headed to the car, another reporter I knew, Catherine Harrop, pulled in. We had a quick chat, and then she told me she had just come from seeing our mutual friend, David Skinner.

In all the excitement, I hadn't been to see him since the previous week, when I met his son at the hospital. I asked how he was doing today and she said not well. He had been moved to hospice care downtown.

I was stunned. His health was gone, as was his luck. He had survived almost two decades past his diagnosis, but there were no more experimental options left for his battered body. I had to go see him immediately. Time was running out.

Meeting Monica after her work, I went right down to the hospice house and spent about an hour with him, just the two of us, as he faded in and out. He knew who I was, which helped me deal with the pain of seeing him fading. He had his guitar there, an old Yamaha like mine, and he got me to play it a little.

He finally said he'd have to lie down, but he was too fatigued to get all the way into bed. I ran and got a nurse and she got him comfortable, then we quietly said our goodbyes and I left, knowing the next time I saw him would probably be at his funeral. It hurt a lot. I so wanted to give Coleen a hug before I left but couldn't as she was out dealing with the fact that his life was coming to an end. There was no more chasing around North America participating in medical experiments to keep him alive like they had done the last twenty-four years. There was a finality to his journey. As we were learning, family caregivers often suffer in silence.

I'm grateful I had so much to focus on I could easily be distracted from the sadness. It was two days from show time; two days from sharing the stage with old bandmates; two days from seeing family, old friends, and fans who hadn't seen us perform in nearly two decades.

Then, one phone call gave me two days of worry and two sleepless nights. It seemed I'd been getting a steady diet of curveballs, which only added to my swallowing issues. A scheduling conflict with the drummer meant he was going to have to choose our show or one in another city, with a country recording artist who had him under contract. I was fuming. We spent two days trying to work it out, but we just couldn't, and then it was gig day and we didn't have a drummer. We needed someone who knew our material, which was almost all original. There was only one drummer in Fredericton who fit that bill.

Somehow, he was available.

Wayne Blanchard saved our asses and graciously said he'd do the show. I sent him the songs, some of which he knew, some of which he had to spend the afternoon learning at home. Wayne hadn't played with us live since 1993, but I knew he was up to the task. The show would go on!

My nerves were nearly shot by noon, not with normal butterflies. I knew we would never be able to pull off what we had rehearsed. Alan and Craig were on their way and didn't even know yet of the drummer change. I called the other two musicians, Dan Robichaud and Dave, and we all agreed to do our best; it's all we could do.

We arrived at the venue early that evening; I knew the other three groups playing and I wanted to see them. Backstage at the tent was always a sweet spot for chatting. Old friends, musicians, and volunteers from my past were all happy to see me back, and surprised I was going to try to perform. Merredith, the stage manager, gave me a huge hug. She missed our working together during HJBF. Between the two of us, we always got the job done, which is not easy when the job is to herd several groups of musicians three nights in a row.

The first act was Quinn Bonnell, the son of another musician friend, Joe Bonnell. He was an up-and-coming artist playing his own songs with a new rock band. He had sat in with us at jams and even one gig. When I needed a drummer and lead player, father and son stepped in, with Quinn on drums.

After their set, it was our turn, so we started to set up. Everyone was there except Wayne, who is well known for arriving just before a gig. I knew he'd be there, but with six minutes to start time, he was cutting it tight!

My close friend Marty and his wife were in the audience. We had been the stage managers during the early years of HJBF, and now Marty was head stage manager on the festival committee. He is also a doctor, my old chiropractor, so he knows me well. He came to a side entrance by the stage and asked if there was a doctor backstage. "Why?" I asked. He said he could see the stress etched deep in my face from halfway back in the audience, and he was genuinely worried I might collapse or worse. I assured him I'd be fine. Besides, my friend Len was watching my every move for Monica. Paramedics were on site. We had a sold-out event, and I wasn't going to miss this for anything! Surely that was clear by now.

Even the stage manager began to wonder if we should call another drummer. I laughed and told her there was no other, that he'd be here or there would be no show at all. Can you imagine just how embarrassing that would have been?

Sure enough, Wayne came in the back entrance just in time, put his cymbals on their stands, put his ear protection on, and picked up the drumsticks, and away we went. Just like old times.

The band started out as a four piece, with two guitars, bass, and drums, as Dan Robichaud and I sat backstage waiting for our turn. Dan is another old friend, fellow educator, and wicked harmonica player who recorded a couple of great tracks with us in the late nineties when he was with the band. We didn't see each other often now, so we were constantly chatting while the show went on. He was going to get up about halfway into the show.

No show is perfect, and this one was far from an exception. During the very first number some missed the outro three times, despite Dave trying to lead them into it, and they had to go around and around before they found a way out.

After the third or fourth tune, Alan's brand-new amp blew up; luckily there was another already there as part of the backline. Unfortunately, he forgot to patch his pedals into the new amp, so there was a change in tone and there was nothing we could do about it.

The crowd was having fun anyway, cheering each time the band finished a tune or solo. It was good to hear the songs live again, but so weird to be backstage and not on it.

It was now time for Dan to be announced. I told him his stage presence was just what we needed and he let me know not to worry. He went up and commanded that stage. He played a couple of killer tunes with some big solos to warm up, adding another dimension to our mix, and the crowd cheered. We were rockin' now, and it sounded better as the set went on. I would slip out from behind to the side stage for some photos every now and then.

Then it was my turn. After telling them to cut a song so we'd keep within time limit, I stumbled to the stage, still dragging my right leg behind me, grabbed my guitar, and then headed for the centre-stage microphone. This was the moment I had worked so hard for, and now it was happening. The adrenaline alone was making me high. A huge roar went up as Dan introduced me with an unscripted, "Ladies and gentlemen, the Miracle Man, Bruce Hughes." In that moment, I knew all the hard work, worry, and tears were going to be worth the next fifteen minutes.

As I started to speak, I noticed Monica with half a dozen of the nurses from 3NE rehab unit right up front, off to my right. I saw Lisa, Heather, Vanessa, Jenna, Allison, and Rebecca. I found out later that Monica had seen them at the back and told them to move up so I'd see them.

I quickly acknowledged them as nurses and how they helped get me here, and they let out an unforgettable shriek of happiness, which was quickly drowned out by the crowd thanking them with their applause. I have it on video and it still gives me chills when I hear it. The nurses were streaming the show for the staff who were working and some of the patients who were pulling for me, too.

So off we went again, now a six-piece band, playing one of our songs, written by Alan, called "Changes," then a cover of Walter Trout's tune "Life in The Jungle"—two of my favourite songs from our past and fitting for that night by title alone! In between songs I talked to the crowd and acknowledged some old faces, like Alan's mom, Shirley, whose house we rehearsed at every Sunday for years.

We saved our best-known song till last.

Of the six songs we had on the local airways back in the nineties, "End of Nowhere" was a fan favourite, a three-chord ditty with an infectious groove. I still play it with The UnHeard, Alan still performs it when he's out playing, and it's still in rotation at a couple local radio stations. I sang lead vocal this time to take us out. We arranged it for crowd participation, Dan egging them on. It was the perfect big ending for our set, in spite of the stumbles to get there.

As the last notes rang out, the crowd gave us one more super round of applause. We gathered centre stage in a line, took a bow, and it was over.

I was thrilled to hear later that for the first time in the festival's history, all five of their major venues sold out on a Friday night. We were up against the heavy-hitter headliners and still managed to fill our venue. That made me proud and so grateful to each and every person that took the time to spend the hour with us. I was truly humbled.

There were two more bands up after us, more old friends in the Gary Sappier Experience and Fredericton's own institution, the Downtown Blues Band, so we hung around talking with musicians, fans, and staff. A few fans who bought our commemorative CDs wanted our autographs. After all the obstacles thrown in our path, it was an awesome night for all the right reasons. I'm a lucky man, but by one o'clock in the morning, I was an exhausted one, too.

We walked back to the car in the parkade a few blocks away, me with a balanced load: guitar in one hand, amp in the other. A friend came up behind me and took my baggage out of my left hand, thinking they'd lighten my load, but I took about ten quick steps sideways to the right before I could regain my balance from the weight shift. (Another lesson all of us survivors know is to only help when we're asked.) It was funny, but it showed me I still had a long way to go. I still walk with something in each hand for balance when I'm gigging.

As we walked down Queen Street, we passed a bar with its large window open and we could hear a band playing inside. I stopped to look—a good spot to rest, anyway—and saw that the guitar player was Greg Webber, who got his start playing with friends at the school where I used to work. He had now become a music teacher himself and fronted his own band, Kill Chicago, playing original material. When I waved, he grabbed at his heart then thumped his chest, sending me love and solidarity. It gave me a boost of energy to get my gear to the car. Monica had to drive us home, of course; I still wasn't as independent as I wanted to be.

At home, I locked the car. Unloading my gear could wait for tomorrow. The night was over, reunion mission complete. Now what? I was hoping for a deep sleep at least.

But, while I needed a couple of days of recovery, I wouldn't get any real rest yet. We heard from Coleen the terrible news that David had passed. His funeral would be at the beginning of the week. Monica and I were so honoured to attend. It gave me a chance to meet more of his friends and his former colleagues from CBC, and I was able to hug Coleen and Lyle again. It was a wonderful service and farewell, and I found myself wishing David could have captured it on camera.

A STROKE OF LUCK

It seems I met David just at the right time, and just in time. Coleen told me he much appreciated the intelligent conversations and the banter we engaged in from the start. For me, David showed me that I had better be my best advocate and to never give up on seeking answers to my medical questions, even if there were none; the journey was about gaining knowledge and not giving up.

David and Coleen also reminded me that no matter how bad things seem, hope is a powerful force.

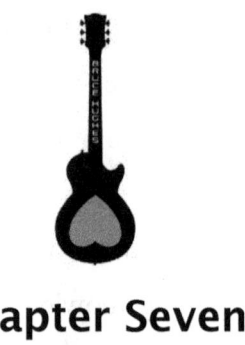

Chapter Seven

Bruce Hughes Should Have Died

Through all of this busyness, I was continuing my outpatient therapy sessions, and they were going well, especially when I got invited to participate in a weekend workshop. It was a clinic for some of the province's physiotherapists to learn the latest or practice new techniques. Two therapists from a Vancouver hospital were the guests, teaching and then supervising the groups. One could see right away I was having trouble with my right leg and foot.

She began to show the group I was assigned to how to break down every toe joint, bending them back and forth, squishing them to force movement. She worked my ankle and knee as well. I was always on the verge of pain, which was obvious to a couple of the therapists, but I hoped it would help my brain and leg working properly together again.

For the next five or six weeks, the head of the physio department, another Lisa, worked on me in the same manner: giving it all a good stretch and then manipulating my toes, ankle, and leg. Then I'd do balance exercises, treadmill, and yoga moves.

I had been dragging my leg around for months now. The leg wasn't working yet—I had no knee bend—but my toes and ankle were getting better, with less numbness and tingling. We carried on with the intense foot manipulation in biweekly outpatient sessions, after the special clinic.

And then one weekend, I went to the field to throw some Frisbee with Willow and bang—my right leg worked. For the first time, I didn't have to drag it or swing it to the side. My knee bent, and the leg followed straight through like it should, just like Maureen and Lisa had reminded me so many times. I couldn't wait to show Monica when she came home from work. I didn't want to sit down, so I continued walking around the field, then down to the river with Willow for a walk on the gravel beds, still using a walking stick in case.

After I regained that leg function, I tried driving again and eventually got my driver's license back. A big day in any stroke survivor's journey, and one that often doesn't come. But I recall the day very well, the day I knew I would be able to drive again. It meant I regained some freedom, more of a sense of myself, again.

I was so incredibly lucky, and I knew it. All I could think about was what I could do to help other stroke survivors. Dr. Bouma and I talked a couple of months earlier about the possibility of doing some major fundraising to bring a medical suite to our hospital that could do the type of procedure that saved me. At the time, only the Saint John hospital offered it, which meant that, with guidelines stating the procedure had to be done within six hours, the travel time alone would prevent some patients from ever benefiting from the procedure. It wasn't right, but that was the reality. More availability might save more lives.

But it turns out, it would cost $3–5 million just to have a suite and equipment. Then you'd have to factor in recruiting staff, recognizing the equipment would be used maybe only once a week, due to the rarity of circumstance and of those who would meet the criteria to have the procedure. I was prepared to do whatever it took to make it happen, but when the practical application and financial reality set in, we had to abandon our noble plan. It bothers me to this day.

Still, I had to do something. From the ashes of failure, a plan B arose. I thought, why not do a massive PR campaign to further educate the public about strokes and how important it is to get help as soon as possible? "Time is brain," Dr. Bouma would always say to me. I knew a lot of local journalists, and I thought I would approach some CBC friends to see if I could garner some interest.

I contacted reporter Catherine Harrop and cameraman Ed Hunter to pitch them on the storyline. They both thought it was a great idea and agreed to pitch it to their superiors. I trusted both of them and knew if there was a chance to do the story, they would make it happen. Boy, did they make it happen! They grabbed on to the "medical Miracle Man" moniker the nurses had given me and ran with it bigtime.

For a full month, Catherine and Ed followed me around, talking to doctors, nurses, and therapists about my case and recovery, all the while getting video footage for a planned TV segment, as well as good soundbites for a radio piece. They were also planning to publish articles online as well.

I had convinced Dr. Bouma to do an interview with Catherine, so she could explain the scientific and technical aspects of my stroke. She was so good at explaining things in terms I could understand, I knew she would be perfect to speak to the public. Dr. Bouma was reluctant and nervous, and was busy with her work, but she still made time for the interview, and she was as good as I anticipated. The interview was set up at her office, and I sat off camera watching while she explained my stroke and recovery using images of my brain scans on her computer screen. She also pushed the need for people to call 911 or get to an emergency room as soon as possible. Too many ignore the signs. "Time is brain," she said again, and commented how my recovery was better than any she had seen for such a severe series of strokes, even agreeing I was "a bit of a Miracle Man." Her voice cracked when she said that, and it seemed tears were close to the surface for everyone in that room.

Catherine and Ed also went to the Saint John Regional Hospital to speak with Dr. Archer, who did my procedure, the endovascular therapy—a thrombectomy, to be precise. They also brought a crew, including my old friend Bill MacDonald, a cameraman, to the outpatient clinic. There Catherine spoke with Maureen and Lisa, the physiotherapists who had worked with me the most.

Last, they did an interview with me at my mom's house on Cherry Avenue in Fredericton, where I lived in my formative years and where I stayed those first few weekends out of hospital. Unfortunately, it was the worst speech day I'd had in a while, and I was slurring my words noticeably—usually a sign I haven't gotten enough sleep.

We set up in the living room, Catherine and I sitting facing each other. Ed had the two cameras framed nicely, with tight shots to capture us up close when talking. We went back and forth for ten minutes or so, though we could have talked for an hour. It was the last piece they needed.

A STROKE OF LUCK

Now Catherine had to write a script to tell my story, and they needed to edit together all the footage to just over two minutes for the TV newscast—a difficult feat with so many elements and so much information, but we all agreed our message was worth all the many weeks of work if it saved even one life or inspired one stroke survivor in their recovery.

A day or two before the full release, Catherine started posting preview videos on the CBC website. Then, on November 20, 2017, all CBC platforms unveiled the Miracle Man story. They published a very detailed online article full of photographs and embedded videos of various interviews. The first line of the article said it all: *Bruce Hughes should have died.* It gave me chills to see that in print, knowing it was true and feeling profoundly thankful to be alive.

You can still find the article on the CBC website: "A Stroke of Luck." It floored me then and still does when I read it again or someone wants to talk about it with me, especially stroke survivors or their caregivers.

On the morning radio show, there was an almost eleven-minute segment covering the whole story. I teared up when I listened to it. People started calling and messaging us; clearly we'd struck a chord.

CBC TV played preview clips all day, and finally at suppertime the provincial TV newscast aired. It helped me so much to see the whole thing put together and explained so well. It was truly the first time I understood what had happened to me and how lucky I was to not only live, but to have such an outstanding recovery. I was in awe.

Catherine somehow managed to convince her colleagues to extend the segment to about three and a half minutes—a proportionally huge chunk of a twenty-two-minute broadcast. I sent thank you notes to Catherine and Ed, asking them to thank everyone else involved in making this campaign happen.

I wanted to publicly thank my massive team of healthcare pros while at the same time getting the FAST (Face, Arm, Speech, Time) public relations message out there. Local media helped me say it all. My story was picked up and shared on social media over a thousand times that first day. Our local paper, *The Daily Gleaner*, called and set up an interview for the next day. Veteran writer Don McPherson asked if we could meet at the hospital so he could also talk to some of those who had worked on me, get some photos and a real sense of the story. I was happy to accommodate if the hospital was, and he took care of the paperwork and requests so we were able to meet and get the job done. His story was published the day after the interview, with the headline *Mind Over Matter*. I often said that was what my recovery felt like; my will to get better, neuroplasticity, and rewiring the brain. Mind over matter.

Another call came from an old friend, Dennis Atchison, to do his YouTube show, *The Dennis Report*. It was an hour at the table, one on one. We went deep on my story and on strokes in general; we also covered music and politics, two other topics we both loved to talk about over the years. It made for a great hour. Dennis had tears in his eyes at times, but we had a blast. Once the show was up there were a couple of thousand views in no time; the message and story were resonating with his audience, too.

My next weekly visit to the hospital was extra special. From the information desk at the front door, past the volunteer desk to the little coffee shop in the lobby, people were commenting on the story. Many of the people I'd been saying hello to every day during my stay didn't know my whole story until they saw it on the news. I reminded them why I was doing all this media—not for me, but to help others who may experience a stroke. Strokes can be devastating and debilitating, when they're not deadly. Odds are that everyone knows someone who will have a stroke, so we should all be prepared.

I went up the elevator to 3NE, and when I rounded the corner I could see a few nurses gathered around their station. They smiled so wide to see me, and we shared big hugs. Some other patients were complimenting me on the story. I've always felt awkward about being the centre of attention, preferring to be a voice or messenger for whatever issue I was discussing in a public setting, and this was no exception. But I could tell everyone was happy for me and proud to have been along for the ride. I got the same greetings and applause on the other two floors I visited that day. I was truly humbled by the love and respect I received from so many. I owed the staff there everything, but they expected nothing; they were just doing what they do—day after day.

Chapter Eight

A Long Winter

In December 2017, word came that a Patient Experience Advisor (PEA) position was mine, if I wanted it. What an honour to represent the patient perspective for therapeutic services. I just had to do it.

Christmas was fast approaching, a time of year I don't care for much. I love Christmas Day, though, and especially the meal, which in recent years was a beautiful turkey dinner at Mom's place. Monica loves it too, and being so far from her family in Edmonton, and with her Dad having passed only a couple of years ago just days before Christmas, I wanted it to be a good one for her. We all needed it.

I went to see my father in Cambridge Narrows. After more than twenty years, we had started talking again. Monica's father's passing made me think about our relationship and I knew Dad would never reach out to me. I would have to initiate contact.

He began drinking decades ago after being a great father to his five children. Liquor got the better of him, like it does so many, ruining his marriage and most of his other relationships too. Even though I was pissed at what he'd done to himself and our family, I still worried about him being at that old farmhouse alone. Monica and I took him some food for gifts and spent a day with him. He didn't look well, and I told him he should go to the doctor or clinic to get checked out.

The best part of Christmas 2017 was the gift my sister, Susan, a talented artist, designed and had printed for me: my very own "Miracle Man" T-shirt. I loved it. It was brilliant, with the shadowy image of my Gibson electric guitar, my name in the fretboard, and a heart upside down in the body to represent how I poured my heart out no matter what I did. She knows me well and had perfectly captured the spirit of events that year.

With the holiday season over, so ended a remarkable 2017, a year that I was grateful to say goodbye to. I welcomed the new year and the possibilities it would bring. It had to be better than the last.

As funny as it sounds coming from someone who shouldn't be here at all, the older I get the more I dislike winter. Winters in New Brunswick are often brutal, and this one was extra nasty. Storm after storm of snow, wind, freezing then thawing—it was a wild one.

Most of my time was spent exhausting myself snow blowing, hauling the snowblower to my friend John's garage for repair, or getting Willow some Frisbee time and exercise. There were a few highlights every week—visiting the hospital as PEA on Tuesdays, and weekly band rehearsals on Sunday. But otherwise winter just felt like a slog.

The PEA role was definitely fascinating. Besides visiting patients and staff in the acute care and rehab units, my PEA duties called for some committee work with their stroke network, sitting in on the odd interview, and some training. It was a huge learning curve in a world I had never thought about but was eager to dive into. At every meeting, I learned something new, especially the jargon; every profession seems to have its own code.

In between these meetings, I managed to help out at a couple of bake sales that 3NE was holding to raise funds for the 11th World Stroke Congress in Montreal. The Congress was coming to Canada for the first time in the fall of 2018. The staff of 3NE had worked hard all year with the plan of taking as many colleagues to Montreal as they could with the money raised for their education fund. It wasn't cheap to send staff away to conferences so they could update their knowledge and skills to apply best practices. Luckily most of the nurses were good bakers, as is Monica, and the people were buying what they were selling! In two sales alone, they raised almost three thousand dollars. I know I ate at least twenty bucks' worth at each.

As good as all that was, Sunday band rehearsals were the best therapy for me. It was so great to see the boys every week, no matter how tired I was. They had stuck with me, a band of brothers helping me learn to play and sing again, to get my rhythm back, maybe my mojo too.

We all knew it would be a long winter without shows, so it gave us the opportunity to write our own music, a dream for any musician and a vision I'd had for this group since we formed. We'd been dabbling with some originals when I had my stroke, and this now gave us the time to really focus on doing that work. In time, we all came to see my misfortune as a blessing…taken from the "when life hands you lemons" file.

One day as we were setting up for a session, Vaughan stopped and came over and gave me a hug. He said, "Every now and then, as we're jamming, I look over and I'm still amazed you're standing there in your spot again." His mother was a former nurse and a big fan of the band. When Vaughan would tell her of my progress, she couldn't believe it either.

We spent the rest of the winter coming up with about fifteen original songs. We had a loose agreement that, with three lead vocalists, whoever wrote the lyrics would sing the song. I wasn't keen on that at first, thinking I could never sing again with my monotone voice, common with strokes, but the boys kept reminding me that it should be part of my continuing speech therapy.

I wouldn't have blamed them if they had scouted another guitar player. There were so many much better than me who would have loved to play with these guys. But they stuck with me, and I didn't want to let them down. Still, I quietly doubted I could keep up, and I didn't want to hold them back.

The boys started bringing some wicked tunes to rehearsals and we'd thrash them out. In no time we were getting almost a full set's worth. I wasn't writing much, focusing more on needing to vastly improve my playing, but one song I penned, "Day After Day," I hope to get recorded and perhaps use in a fundraising campaign someday. It's a great little three-chord rocker that the boys dressed up nicely with their parts. Vaughan even wrote a killer lead break for it. The song is a three-minute ride on my stroke journey, paying tribute to those who got me through it all. I owe them my life. The least I could do was write a song for them.

DAY AFTER DAY

    Waiting for the sun to rise
    To brighten up the day
    Waiting on an angel of mercy
    To help me find my way

Tell me why I'm living this way
Night after night, day after day
Sun goes down
And the moon comes up
Hope begins to fade
Sleepless nights and endless doubts
Drown the cries of pain
Tell me why I'm living this way
Night after night, day after day
Healing hands and a lot of love
Soon I was on my way
Ashes to ashes, dust to dust
Await our dying days
Tell me why I'm living this way
Night after night, day after day
Tell me why we're living this way
Night after night, day after day

We couldn't wait for the summer to come so we could go play some of these songs in public for the first time and hopefully get some recorded later. We were on to something special, we could feel it, and the band was getting tighter all the time. Every week it seemed a song or two would take shape. The other three guys worked full-time and did not have a lot of free time on their hands, with their responsibilities and raising families. This was their therapy, too. I continued to try and get as much coordination as I could back between my brain and hands, a very slow process this far out from my strokes, but small improvements emerged from time to time, spurring me on.

Later in February, I received a call from someone assuming I had done another interview with CBC, as they had seen a segment on the provincial TV news that night. I rarely missed watching the show but had that night. I said I hadn't interviewed lately, that maybe they just did a rerun of my story or something like that, but I'd check it out online.

I discovered CBC had done a piece condensing my story to lead into the major medical announcement breaking that day, that the Heart and Stroke Foundation of Canada's guideline for tPA and endovascular therapy would be recommended to be extended from the previous six hours to now twenty-four hours.

I had gone nine hours without blood flow to my brain and proven it could all be done safely with a good recovery. My case helped medical professionals build theirs to open the window. It was estimated that potentially two or three hundred more people every year could be saved from death or major debilitation. (Sadly, after more testing, it was later determined that Heart and Stroke may rescind the recommendation, as evidence failed to produce the desired results. Maybe I really am a freak.) After playing the news clip for Monica, I vowed to track down the two doctors at Saint John Regional Hospital who performed the procedure on me, Dr. Brain Archer and Dr. Jake Swan. I had always wanted to meet and thank them but hadn't yet had the chance.

Coming into spring, I continued my weekly visits at the hospital, stopping by the 3NE rehab unit and often seeing someone I knew or had met the week before in the 4NW acute stroke care unit. Too often I saw someone I knew or parents of friends having extended stays for whatever reason. Knees and hip replacements were common, but the stroke survivors and families were my focus.

There is a never-ending need for rehabilitation services, in a province with the oldest population per capita and no sign of the government increasing resources to meet increasing demands. I would love to see more therapists working full-time, getting patients healthier faster and out the door to independent living or at least more satisfying lives in a suitable home. It bothers me that the therapists don't get replaced if they are sick or otherwise unable to work on a given day. It is crucial in recovery to get the required therapy. As a patient, it pissed me off to no end to have a session cancelled.

*

In March, I learned that Dave, my old friend and bass player in Blind Dog, had had a heart attack and was scheduled for open heart surgery as soon as possible. I called him immediately and found out he had some type of tumour on the inside of one of his heart chambers and they'd have to crack him open to get it out. While they were in there, they would clean one clogged artery as well.

The surgery went well, but at times he had an irregular heartbeat, so it took a while to figure out. I spoke with Dave a few times during his ordeal, and we both realized how lucky we were to not only have good healthcare and support to recover so well, but also to have been able to play the reunion show. As the years go by, you can't afford to wait, it seems. Dave fully recovered and is back doing the two things he enjoys the most—playing bass and playing golf. He's great at both.

March continued to live up to its billing as the cruellest month. Another old friend passed away; one I had visited many times in hospital in recent months. I'd known Ann since she was in grade eight at Albert Street Junior High and I was in grade ten at Fredericton High School. I knew her children, too. She was a sweetheart who had been fighting ill health for decades and finally succumbed to its ravages.

She and her daughter sent me a photo, with Ann flashing a peace sign the day before she passed. At least I got to share the grief with her family and friends at her funeral. While there, I met a relative of hers who worked on a boat from Deer Island that my Dad wrote a song about back in the early sixties called "Fairhaven Queen."

It was just the beginning of a flood of people I knew who died over the next few months. Almost every week there was another funeral or visitation, half of them younger than I. Such a shame! I never seemed to get over the shock of one loss before another would smack me down. It took its toll on me emotionally. So much sorrow, so many hurting. My PEA role and band rehearsals couldn't come fast enough to distract me and relieve some stress. It had been a long winter.

April showers might bring May flowers in most places, but in New Brunswick we get April flooding. This year brought a record spring freshet and flood, devastating many people and properties from Fredericton south to the Bay of Fundy. Our property on the Keswick River saw substantial damage, with major land erosion of about fifteen feet, instead of the usual foot or so. It undercut the bank so much that our twelve-by-twenty-foot garage fell into the river, and after about five hours of sitting in the water like it was in a giant wringer washer, it exploded and floated away in pieces. The swollen river was still cutting through the bank like a hot knife through butter, with only a sandy wall to slow it. My stress levels were off the charts. I had twice attempted to enter a private-public partnership with either the province or federally or both, and I applied for any climate change funding from Ottawa, but all to no avail.

A STROKE OF LUCK

Through all of the loss and anxiety, I was trying to stay focused on a big honour coming my way: I was scheduled to give the stroke survivor speech at the annual New Brunswick stroke conference in Fredericton on May 2, 2018, just shy of a year since my strokes. I was looking forward to sharing my story of never giving up and thanking the many healthcare professionals who helped me get back to a decent quality of life.

The night before my speech there was a public meeting with a Q and A to follow. Monica and I thought we would go, as we still had some questions about my case and our future. It was there I met Dr. Dylan Blacquiere, whom I had seen make the announcement about the possible guideline changes on CBC TV news in February. I had to meet him and pick his brain, to see if I could learn anything more about my case or similar ones, even though they were rare. He was a great speaker and really could explain things well to the audience.

Unfortunately, when I asked my questions, I didn't get helpful answers. Dr. Blacquiere said, "In your case we just don't know." I had gotten used to that brutally honest response; apparently, I *was* the new data. I was pleased to learn medical professionals were using endovascular therapy a little more now and the mortality rate was going down in stroke patients that met the criteria for a thrombectomy, as they refined the procedure.

But only 10–15 percent of strokes met the criteria for endovascular therapy, and still no one had recovered as well as I had. I was so thankful for my life and recovery so far, but not knowing how or why I'd done so well created its own anxiety. It was hard on the head. Every time I had neck pain, especially on the side with the stent, I would automatically worry something was wrong and wonder if this time I wouldn't be so lucky.

After another sleepless night fretting about the flooding and erosion, Monica and I were off to give my speech to start the day's stroke conference.

I had given up on writing any kind of formal speech and instead opted for another idea I had, using photos I had taken during my time in the hospital, from the patient's point of view. I called it "50 Shades of Stay," which drew laughter from the hundreds of healthcare participants in the room. I had a flash drive and they had projection capabilities. So, it was a show-and-tell speech, and I had twenty minutes to fill.

I showed a series of photographs and explained a piece of my journey or how the person in the photo had helped me along my way. From healthcare professionals to family and friends, I tried to show that even though nurses were calling me the Miracle Man, there was a huge team behind me that got me to where I was that day. I owed them all my life and a very public thank you.

The entire presentation was an emotional roller coaster for Monica, and for the many audience members who had been a part of my recovery and journey. From sombre moments to laughter and then tears, the crowd rode right along with me, frame after frame triggering more memories. Sometimes I would call on one of the nurses or therapists to help me recall some detail.

There was no clock on the podium so I had no idea of the time; I figured someone would let me know when mine was up. I just kept talking until I got through all fifty photos, concluded my message, and thanked everyone.

I was stunned at the standing ovation I received from the huge crowd. I could feel my face turn red, having always been shy to be acknowledged, but it did feel good eventually. Monica had tears streaming down her face, proud of me for the speech and for the last year of recovery. One of the chairmen of the conference made a few remarks and presented me with a gift, and then it was time for the next speaker.

I went to our table, gave Monica a kiss, and sat down to hear, "Well, that will be hard to follow," and also something about getting "back on track." I asked for the time and someone at the table told me.

I'd talked for thirty-five minutes!

The next speaker was Dr. Patrice Lindsey, from Toronto, who was not only a knowledgeable stroke doctor and researcher but had also had a stroke herself at the age of thirty-eight. I was fascinated by how she so matter-of-factly discussed where we were in the world of strokes. For example, overall, the new research showed that women were having more devastating strokes and at older ages, but two-thirds of the current research were findings on men.

She discussed the possible new guidelines Dr. Blacquiere had talked about the night before, hoping they could be enacted someday. She had a wealth of information and experience and was a forceful spokesperson in the medical advocacy and public relations fields. I was very impressed with her, as was the rest of the audience.

At the coffee break, we left the main room for the hallway and I got to talk to some of the local nurses and therapists there. Many I knew had come to hear my speech and said how it moved them to hear my side of the journey, one they had witnessed and intervened in firsthand. Other folks I had never met approached to congratulate me or ask questions about my recovery, as they also were a survivor or had a family member in recovery. It was heartwarming and overwhelming, such an outpouring of compassion, but I shouldn't have been surprised. I have deep respect for what these professionals do day after day, even aside from what they did for me personally.

One lovely young woman approached me with a big smile and introduced herself as Moira Teed. She too wanted to congratulate me on my recovery and speech. She was from

Fredericton originally and her parents still lived here, which explained why she looked familiar.

After a decade working at a hospital in Ottawa, she now worked for the national Heart and Stroke Foundation there, in charge of their lived experience program. She and Dr. Lindsay were interested in talking to me about joining a national panel that reviewed stroke guidelines. As participants on the panel, they were including the patient perspective in their considerations and needed a representative from New Brunswick. I was floored and honoured to be considered, and I asked for some more information as to the position and its expectations.

Later, in the next break, Moira and Dr. Lindsay offered me a panel position on the spot. It wouldn't take much of my time—just an hour every three weeks. I would be teleconferencing with survivors and caregivers, discussing our experiences in hopes of improving the quality of care and life of those impacted. I looked forward to it.

As the afternoon sessions wound down, a note made its way to me from someone sitting at our table, though I wasn't sure who. She had seen my red face earlier and heard I was a bit distraught for going so far over my allotted time. Ask anyone who knows me, especially the boys in the band, I don't have much of a poker face, so reading me is easy! She wanted me to know I shouldn't worry about it. Her note said something like, "If anyone should go over their time limit, it's the person giving the survivor speech, and in my opinion your speech was the best of the day!" I looked around the table until I saw a smiling face acknowledging they'd sent the note. I nodded and mouthed a thank you. It sure made me feel better and it capped an exhausting but informative day.

*

Now it was time to return to the daily grind, which at this time was a nightmare, twenty-four hours a day for the foreseeable future.

As bad as the weather was in April, May was even more devastating, with two straight weeks of the worst flooding New Brunswick had ever seen. Rivers and lakes had become one giant pool of water all heading south, trying to squeeze out the narrow rock passage at the end of the Saint John River to the Atlantic Ocean, in the Bay of Fundy—home of the world's highest tides.

So many homes and cottages, businesses, and roads were destroyed or damaged. We at least are still in our home, which is in dire need of some major upgrades that have been put on hold due to both of our health issues.

And May continued to bring tough goodbyes. My good friend Sam, whom I met and had become so close to while we were in rehab, passed away only a few days after my speech. I had just attended his seventieth birthday that winter and met many more of his extended family, as well as old friends. We were unable to attend his funeral service in New Denmark, but Monica and I did go to the visitation in Fredericton to be with his family. His wife, Nancy, is a lovely woman, with an awesome family. We knew we would remain friends.

Within days, I received yet more bad news. Another childhood friend had dropped dead, having had a massive heart attack while out of the country on vacation. When one of the old gang from our schooldays passes, a shockwave goes through our large group of friends. Knowing he died in another country made it even sadder, and, after much delay, a funeral was held and a large turnout of our crowd showed up to pay their respects, to be with his wife and family.

When the service and reception were over, some of us hung out in the parking lot, having a beer and sharing stories or just catching up. I hadn't seen some of the folks in over thirty years. I asked if we could get a group photo and we did: sixteen old friends in one shot, a treasure I shared with his wife.

Later that month, on the same day, mothers of three of my old friends were buried. I wanted to go to all of the funerals, but of course I couldn't, so I ended up going with my mother to the funeral of one of her best friends, Joy. She was also the mother of my best female friend growing up, Kris, who had passed away a couple of summers earlier. Kris had been like a sister to me. Her passing hurt a lot and still does.

I was surrounded by death and tragedy, it seemed; maybe it's the price of knowing so many people. But something had to give. It seemed there was only one thing now that could make me smile and forget the onslaught: music.

*

I was so grateful that Vaughan, Bob, and Charles spent the winter and spring helping rehab my hands and voice. My playing still sucked, but by May I had written a couple of decent tunes to go with the plethora of great ones they were bringing to the table. By the summer, I figured I'd be ready for us to return to playing live, long sets of mostly our own material.

We applied to many festivals and outdoor venues, and we were fortunate to get four or five shows over the summer, thanks to a local production company that had shows booked all around the province. They really liked our band and the material we were writing, and they would help The UnHeard get heard! We had worked some shows in the past with JEM Productions and they always had a nice stage with great gear and technicians, a real pleasure.

We couldn't wait to get our songs out there. Though we'd been building a good following before my stroke, we'd been playing mostly cover songs. How would crowds respond to our originals?

A STROKE OF LUCK

Before the summer festival season was upon us, we decided to go to a local bar on their Wednesday jam night and road test seven of the new songs we had written. It was also a chance for me to test myself.

Dolan's Pub allowed us to use their stage and PA for a forty-minute set. Usually there were only ten to twenty people there for their Wednesday night jam, a shame as the house band was always good, no matter the lineup. But this night over a hundred people showed up, many of them musicians and friends who were itching to see what we had cooked up over the winter. The owner, Barry, messaged me the next day saying what a great night of sales he'd had for a Wednesday. We didn't play our best, we had some little stumbles, but any night on a stage playing new original material beats not playing.

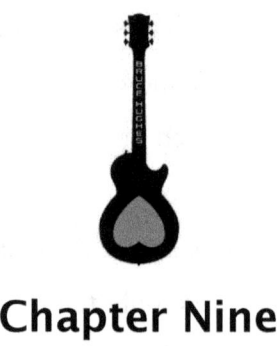

Chapter Nine

Dad

On the May long weekend, Monica, Willow, and I decided to pay another visit to my father to see how he'd fared over the winter. We'd talked a couple of times on the phone and sent emails since Christmas, and I could tell he wasn't doing well, but I had to see him in person.

It wasn't a pretty sight.

Dad had fallen down the stairs that winter and damaged his shoulder, but rather than going to a hospital, he'd just sat there in his chair, watching FOX News and old movies, waiting for it to heal on its own. When he laughed at how dumb Trump supporters must be to believe him, I knew Dad still had at least some mental capacity to have his own opinions and to make his own decisions, even if they were often poor.

A STROKE OF LUCK

It was obvious there was much more wrong with him than just a fall down the stairs. He had lost weight, could barely get around, and even though it was a hot day he wore a heavy black leather jacket on the short walk we took down to the old wharf and back. He looked and sounded terrible.

Again, I told him to get to a doctor, offering to take him, but he said he was waiting for the results of some bloodwork he'd had done at the local clinic. That at least made me feel a little better, that he had done something, so we went home after our visit with him. What he didn't say, as I learned later, was that he'd had the bloodwork done about a year ago.

*

Summer was almost here, the sun's warmth almost able to heal all that ailed me. My aches and pains lessened. Festival season was upon us and I was getting more exercise. Our band's drummer, Charles, gave me a lawnmower with no motor, the push type. At first, I could barely do twenty minutes without being exhausted and my legs feeling like rubber.

A couple of neighbours offered to do the lawns for me, but I insisted I could and needed to do it myself. I used to be able to mow our field in an hour, at most seventy-five minutes, all in one shot. The first time I tackled it this year, it took me three separate sessions over a two-day period. I had a lot of work to do to get as healthy as

I needed to be. I needed more strength and stamina to have any hope of playing the long sets we had lined up.

My other main exercise came from river walks or playing Frisbee with Willow. She seemed to know making me chase her to get it back was good for my development, even though it drove me mad sometimes. She'd rarely drop the Frisbee at my feet as asked; she always placed it just out of reach, or she would make me take it from her.

As I felt my strength growing, I still wasn't sure about whether I could stand with a heavy guitar around my neck for long periods of time, in the heat at that. You don't know until you try, as they say, so I figured to be safe I would buy a little folding stool for the side of the stage that I could use if I felt weak-kneed at any time. A smart crutch, I called it.

The first big gig of the summer was the annual Ribfest in Fredericton on the Exhibition Grounds. A four-day event that drew almost one hundred thousand people, with teams barbecuing, vying to be voted "best ribs." Throw in live music every night and you've got a recipe for fun—just what the doctor ordered in my books.

We had a ninety-minute set, and while we wanted to debut more of our new songs, we didn't have all of them rehearsed well enough to fill the whole time, so we included four or five covers to start with. We planned to get warmed up, give the sound engineers a chance to dial us in, and then do a dozen of our tunes to finish the night. We had a beautiful big stage and a large crowd chomping at the bit, and we couldn't wait to get going!

After our halfhearted cover tunes, we finally launched into our own songs and brought a whole different energy to the show. We kicked it up a notch and the crowd could feel it. There were plenty of little fumbles, but I think only we noticed, because the response from the audience was awesome. One of the sound technicians recorded most of the set off the board. It was dry and you could hear every mistake, but I was happy to have some reference points, so I could get these songs burned into my new brain.

I didn't retain things like before. Being a rhythm player, I used to be able to recall chord progressions of most songs after running through them just a couple of times. Now I had to play along to them at home, over and over, then rehearse them on Sundays with the guys. In spite of it all, the songs were well received, and the sound crew, who were hearing them for the first time as well, really liked them. Always a good sign.

I told little stories in between songs about my recovery and how thankful I was for all the support I had received from everyone. I said how grateful I was to the boys in the band for all of their help and support. A nurse or two who cared for me happened to be there as well. I always had to thank them!

A new friend I'd met at the reunion show the previous fall, Jing, was a really good photographer and captured many nice photos that evening. She sent them to us once she returned back home in Prince Edward Island. We were thrilled she captured us in our element.

It's hard to describe, but there is nothing quite like standing on a stage playing your own songs and having them well received. Not the polite smattering of a few hands, but genuine applause. It is nerve-wracking, but when it works, it's magical. We had found our mojo, and best of all, I didn't need to use my little stool—the adrenaline kept me on my feet the whole set! My playing still had a ways to go, but I sang lead on three or four songs and backup on some others, so all in all it was a successful start to the festival season for The UnHeard. We were back.

Up next, we had a special Canada Day show in Oromocto, New Brunswick, as part of their annual "Pioneer Days." Another ninety-minute set, to which we would add another original song or two. Some of the 3NE nurses were supposed to be attending, and I told the boys I would like to make a little speech and dedicate the new song "Day After Day" to them. I couldn't wait to play it for them and hoped they would like it. We had a couple weeks to prepare, and we wanted to have even more originals ready. There would be no more covers if we could help it. I loved the idea of creating, not covering, and that was the goal of The UnHeard.

A STROKE OF LUCK

*

With summer in full swing, I was enjoying time outside, visiting friends, going to open-air concerts in various city parks, and taking my usual river walks with Willow. All of these were good rehab, physically and mentally, and much needed after such a tough spring.

I decided to go visit my father again, see how he was doing. The old farmhouse was a great spot to be in the summer. I wanted to work in a visit with an old friend I'd considered my best since we were fourteen years old, playing on the same school basketball team. Ted had a summer place on another small lake nearby just off the highway to Dad's. I hoped to stop in to see Ted and his wife, Kathy, whom I had known since she was in grade five, on my way home.

I loaded up and headed out with Willow to go see Dad. When we arrived, the beauty of the day and place quickly took a back seat to my father's appearance. He didn't look or sound well at all.

I'd brought some soup and baking that Monica made for him, knowing he probably wasn't eating well. After a short chat we had something to eat. He wolfed down some soup and a sandwich for lunch in his TV room in front of FOX and CNN news, which were taking turns blaring away while he laughed at them every now and then.

He always appreciated good food, as he had been eating his own modest cooking for decades now and burned most things he made due to setting the stove or burner only on high. He'd ruined more pots and pans than anyone I've ever known and spoiled many meals.

I couldn't get over how much weight he had lost, his shortness of breath, and his skin discoloration. It looked yellow. I asked if he had been to the doctor or clinic like he'd said he would during our last visit in May. He said he still hadn't heard back about the bloodwork and was waiting for their call.

He wasn't helping his own cause, it appeared to me, and I told him he should go get a full examination, perhaps at a hospital in Saint John or Oromocto. He finally admitted he didn't feel well and his mind wasn't as sharp these days.

I stayed most of the day, then headed for home almost feeling guilty. I didn't have a good feeling at all about his situation and decided I'd call my brother Kevin when I got home to see if he had seen Dad lately. If he had, surely, he'd noticed how sick Dad was.

I made my pit stop at Ted and Kathy's summer place. It was always good to see them, and in such a peaceful setting. Every New Brunswicker knows of such a place, even if they don't own one. The "Picture Province," indeed.

Ted was one of my few friends who still had both parents living. Given we turned sixty this year, that put it all in perspective. We weren't kids anymore ourselves. I shared my concern about Dad's health, but Ted and Kathy knew Dad and his stubbornness.

Willow and I headed for home after a couple of hours. It wasn't long on the highway again and she was fast asleep in the back seat. She'd had a "big dog day," as we say. But mine wasn't over yet. I still had to call Kevin.

When I got home, I updated Monica, she headed for bed, and I phoned Kevin. He had regular contact with Dad. He and his son, Kyle, often spend the weekend with him. Surely Kevin had seen the deterioration of Dad's health.

When I called, though, he didn't seem alarmed. After all, Dad was turning eighty-six next week. I told him it was more than just old age, and that Dad admitted his mind was not sharp and he was still waiting on bloodwork. I asked Kevin to go visit Dad soon, and to take Joanne with him; maybe Dad would listen to a nurse telling him to go to the doctor. Kevin said he'd go right away and get back to me. He had a better chance of convincing Dad to do something than I did; their relationship was much closer.

I also mentioned that our band was playing soon in Oromocto. It would be Kevin's best chance to see us live, as it was only half an hour or so from Dad's, if he happened to be visiting Dad that day. Kevin loved music and I knew he would like us.

In no time, July 1, the big Canada Day show in Oromocto, was upon us. The venue was a carnivalesque environment with a covered bandstand in the middle of it all. Good thing. It was a hot and sticky day, so we were glad to have shade. We were playing a few covers and then rolling out our own material. Another crowd to impress, although smaller. Some new fans to make. We had only played in Oromocto once before, at a benefit in their Legion, so we weren't well-known there.

Three of the nurses from my rehab days were sitting with Monica. My friend Dave, the retired pilot, was there. Kevin arrived shortly after we started. I was really glad to look out and see him there. He hadn't seen me perform since the nineties and hadn't seen The UnHeard at all. He was a very good singer in his youth and always loved music, so I knew he was going to really enjoy tonight's show.

After acknowledging him in the audience, I began my little speech and dedication to the nurses and all the healthcare professionals who helped me get to that stage. Then we launched into "Day After Day." One of the nurses, Rebecca, took some video that evening, including that song. Rebecca, Heather, and Jenna loved it and it made me feel good to see them swell with pride.

I got a couple of photos with Kevin. He loved the band and was blown away with our musicianship and original songs. I knew he would be. When we got a moment alone, he told me he had taken Dad to the Oromocto hospital for tests on Friday and they would have results of the new bloodwork on Monday. I was so glad Dad finally did something and I thanked Kevin for getting him there.

A STROKE OF LUCK

*

Throughout the summer I continued to make my weekly visits to the hospital, meeting with rehab patients the staff thought might need their spirits lifted or to talk to someone. Hope is everything in recovery. Not everyone will recover as well as I have, but seeing the real thing in person has had a positive impact on several occasions already.

In addition, I had my PEA committee duties, my national Heart and Stroke Foundation stroke review panel, and many healthcare groups inviting me to speak with their employees or colleagues.

One group I spoke with consisted of managers and directors of departments within the healthcare system. I got to watch and listen much of the day before my time came to speak. An impressive bunch from all over the province, doing what they could to make the healthcare system better—a tough, thankless task at the best of times.

We were divided into smaller groups at times, and activities helped us to get to know each other better. That was always a good thing in my books. We had some lunch and some time outside the meeting facility, watching the ducks in the pond and enjoying the opportunity to have non-shop-related conversations with other attendees.

By mid-afternoon it was my turn to address the crowd and I began another rendition of my "50 Shades of Stay" speech. Maybe I was a bit intimidated by the audience or maybe I was just off that day, but I stumbled through, receiving warm applause anyhow. Each time I speak, I add a photo or say something more, as the original was based on my stay in the hospital. Now it is more than that, much more. It has become a story of hope, not just thanking everyone. I add photos and stories to fit each crowd I speak to, as it isn't always healthcare pros.

Some participants came to me at the next coffee break asking if I could come to their hospital and speak with staff or patients. It is always an honour to be asked to do anything like that if regulations allow. My director of therapeutic services, Patti, was a big supporter of my PEA position, as well as what I did in it. We both like to push boundaries and the line forward, especially for better patient experience and healthcare.

Monica came at the end of the day to pick me up, just as we were loading the cars with all the equipment and supplies needed for the day's outing. Willow was in the car too, but only for another split second, as she either heard my voice or saw the ducks and jumped out the car window and started running around. I heard the commotion and saw Willow completely ignoring Monica's commands. Monica had forgotten a leash, which we usually put on

Willow before she gets out of the car in new places, for exactly this reason.

So after my speech about how my brilliant dog saved my life, neither of us could get her to listen to us at all! It was too funny to be embarrassing, and anyway she came back soon and we got her into the car. Life is humbling sometimes, but it was overall another feel-good day that ended in laughter on the ride home.

*

I really enjoyed working with the national panel review. I always learned something working with Moira and Dr. Lindsay's group of healthcare professionals, fellow survivors, and caregivers who were creating recommendations for best practices stroke guidelines. These guidelines were reviewed every two years, and I was late joining the group, which had recruited me after my speech in the spring. We teleconferenced every three weeks and we had some discussion around the recommended new guidelines announced in February (moving from six to twenty-four hours for tPA and endovascular therapy), as well as brand new and somewhat devastating data from a study on women and strokes. Outcomes are overall much worse for women than men.

Being on this committee was also another chance to hear how other patients and staff dealt with the impacts of strokes and to realize, once again, how lucky I was to be alive and doing so well.

My recovery was remarkable, even according to fellow survivors who had been recovering for much longer. I was just over a year from something that should have killed or at least permanently debilitated me, and here I was walking and talking again, with maybe 20 percent of my recovery to go.

*

A couple of days after the Canada Day show Kevin came to, he called me with an update on Dad's bloodwork. Apparently Dad got a call on the weekend asking him to return as soon as possible to do further tests for a proper diagnosis. We worried whether Dad would even bother going, knowing what a procrastinator he was. Luckily, Kevin managed to get him to go, doing his grocery shopping for him while he was at the Oromocto hospital for bloodwork. Within another day or two Kevin called me again. Kevin had taken Dad in for his results, and they were not good.

Dad was full of cancer. His lungs, lymph nodes, and liver were all in bad shape. That certainly explained the yellowish hue he'd had for the last few weeks. They were giving him four to six months to live, but in my gut I didn't think he would make it even that long.

I asked Kevin if they admitted him to hospital. He said they gave him the choice to stay in hospital or to go home. Of course, Dad was scared and wanted to go home, and Kevin didn't fight him on it, even though we knew him staying in hospital would be better for us all.

Kevin left his job to stay at Dad's place and provide care for him there. There was some compassionate care program he may be able to tap into to cover some costs, but the emotional toll can never be quantified. Still, we couldn't blame Dad for wanting to die at home.

After talking with Kevin, I called Joanne, who had seen Dad recently. We always talked openly and honestly about everything, no secrets and no topics out of bounds. I hoped to get some straight medical answers from her about Dad based on her experiences as a nurse. The first thing I asked about was the idea that Dad had four to six months to live. Was this just a standard way of preparing family for someone's death, or was it a plausible timeline for Dad specifically? Joanne said basically it was a standard message; she agreed with me after seeing Dad and his latest bloodwork results that he more likely had four to six weeks, not months. His time was running out—fast.

For the next two weeks Dad stayed at Kevin's place, with Kevin doing what he could to feed and care for him. There were constant phone calls between us, and a couple more day trips for Willow and me to see them. Dad could barely breathe or stay awake these days and it was hard to watch.

On one trip, Dad offered to give me his first guitar, an old Zen-On six string he got for his twelfth birthday from his older brother Jimmy. That would have been 1944 if his recollection was right. The guitar was in rough shape, but I told him I'd take it to a luthier to see if it could be repaired to play again. I had seen it kicking around various closets over the years but I didn't know it was his first guitar. That made it a real treasure to me, regardless of its financial value.

Then one day, Kevin called and said that Dad had talked with the doctor again and agreed it was time to go to the palliative care unit in the Saint John Regional Hospital. We were all relieved, as strange as that may sound. The end was near, but at least he'd be in a better setting. After he settled in I would go to see him. Kevin and Joanne and our sister, Susan, all lived closer to the hospital, and they could keep a daily check on him.

Within a couple of days, Monica and I headed for our first (and second-last) visit with Dad in the Saint John Regional Hospital. Both Dad and I had a fear of hospitals, but I had gotten over mine after having my strokes. I had a whole new outlook on hospitals and was hoping Dad did, too, now that he saw how helpful staff were, how vital the care was.

Turns out he did. Between his laboured breaths, we had a great chat about how well he was being cared for and how much he liked his room, which was like an apartment, he thought. I was so glad to see him comfortable in his surroundings.

His only complaints were that he was always itchy, which they were giving him meds for but never enough, it seemed, and that he had to have assistance to go to the washroom, as he was a fall risk. Nothing more they could do about the itching other than meds, and at least he wasn't on a catheter yet. But again, I knew having that bit of bathroom dignity matters to the patient.

After some time he was tired and less talkative, nodding off a bit. I thought I'd let him rest and I would go for a little walk to get some sunshine and fresh air. Monica would stay with him, as my siblings said he didn't like to wake up and see no one there. He was still scared.

After a few hours, other family members began to arrive for their daily visits. Dad grabbed my hand as I was leaving and started to tremble and cry a little. I knew it was his way of telling me he loved me, and I was hoping he realized what we had lost by not having a relationship for so long. We had just started to talk again in the last couple of years and now he was going to die before we could come close to repairing our damaged relationship. It was a harsh lesson for us both that I hope others never have to learn. We don't get do-overs.

Monica and I headed for home and said we'd return to visit on her next days off. It was hard for us, with one car and Monica working again. We couldn't go visit every day so we'd do what we could.

On the way home Monica told me a very important moment she had with Dad while I left the room earlier for some air. She said Dad apologized to her for treating her badly back when he and I stopped talking. She didn't deserve to be caught in the crossfire all those years, but then again, neither did my mom or sister. I think Dad had a problem with smart, independent women. I call it the fifties mentality—the idea that women should be barefoot and pregnant. Homemakers, not homeowners.

I was shocked but so happy to hear he'd apologized. To admit to himself he was wrong was one thing; to say it to her was another. I wish I'd been there when he apologized, but at least he did—to one of us, anyway. Monica felt good about it, and that was the most important thing for me.

In just a few days, the call came that we needed to come as soon as possible if we wanted to talk with him or see him once more. Our good friends Rowena and Danny were taking care of Willow when we had to travel, so we knew we could take our time on this trip if necessary.

What a difference a few days made. Dad was now bedridden, barely speaking or conscious. He did manage to recognize and acknowledge us. He was still itchy and always thirsty, and about all he could take in were liquids. His doctor and a nurse were scheduled to stop by for a final meeting with him and any family that could come. They were so kind.

Dad thanked them for their care and the nurse said what a model patient he had been—something we never thought we'd hear. After the meeting and some more water and meds, Dad began to doze off again, so I thought I'd go for a walk around the hospital to see if by chance either of the doctors who'd worked on me during my lifesaving endovascular therapy were working today so I could finally thank them or at least leave a message.

Off I went, without any idea where to look. I'd been in this hospital a few times when I was looking after Kevin and Joanne after their surgeries, but it was a huge complex and mostly unfamiliar to me. All I knew was that Dr. Archer and Dr. Swan were interventional radiologists, so I followed some signs that led me to the X-ray area and eventually found a woman at a desk to ask if she knew of the doctors I was looking for.

It turns out she worked for them—this was their office. Both doctors were in that day, but at the moment they were in the middle of a procedure similar to the one they'd performed on me. She said she hoped I could come back later and that they would love to see me. Everyone there seemed to know my story or recognize me.

I told her about being in the palliative care unit with my father, and it turned out she was good friends with my brother's son, Kyle. She had seen Kevin and Joanne visiting Dad that week. She said she'd text one of them when the doctors were ready to see me. I went back to Dad's room and told my family about the connection. At least there was something positive in my world today.

In about an hour, I got the text. I had seen Dr. Archer's face before in the CBC News report but had never seen Dr. Swan. Still in their scrubs and one holding a coffee, they met me in the hallway. They both looked so young, and they couldn't have been nicer. They said they almost never got to meet the people they worked on, let alone hear of such a great recovery from such a devastating series of rare strokes.

They were amazed at how well I could walk and talk, how my cognitive skills were virtually intact. They took me to the room where they'd performed the procedure on me, showed me more 3D movies of the actual procedure, and made copies for me.

I asked, "What made you think of using a heart stent to repair the torn brain stem artery?" It was then I learned I was not the first but the second patient to have the procedure tried in this way. About a month prior to me, a patient in PEI had been saved by a similar procedure, but apparently he hadn't recovered as well as me.

After they'd answered every question they could and given me more than enough of their time, I thanked them—not only for only saving me, but also for what they did every day. They are real heroes to me and I'm sure to many others.

They insisted on getting a photo of the three of us, which they would forward to me later in the day. I was thrilled and proudly stood in the middle with my arms around them both. Their smiles couldn't have been any bigger or more genuine. It made our day, all of us. I wish more people could meet face to face and thank those who've saved their lives or helped heal them in other ways.

I would have to savour that feeling later, though; for now, I left to go back to Dad's room and that reality.

He was barely conscious for more than a minute or two at a time now before falling back to sleep. It was getting late, and two of my siblings had arrived for the night, so Monica and I said our goodbyes to Dad, gave him a kiss on the forehead, and left.

It was a long drive home that night wondering if it would be our last time seeing him, knowing it probably was.

I had a PEA meeting in the next couple of days at our hospital, so I was able to get my mind off Dad for a while, but within a day or two the call came that he was being put on morphine to help ease him into the big sleep. The next day, July 26, 2018, he passed. It was less than four weeks from the bloodwork that showed he was full of cancer, just as Joanne and I anticipated. He had a very rapid decline, and while it's heartbreaking, it might also be a blessing.

Kevin and Susan would handle all the arrangements and get Dad cremated, then figure out what to do. He didn't want a funeral. Susan said she talked to him and he just wanted to have his ashes put in an old can from his house in Cambridge-Narrows. She decided to take care of that. Kevin was made executor of his will and estate—probably not an easy task, knowing our father; he wasn't great with paperwork. Kevin would no doubt be busy for some time.

It was sad, but it was over, and I had to find a way to deal with it. As I had stated to some close friends, I had sorrow but no pity. I found it hard to feel bad for someone who'd done that much harm to himself and to his most important relationships. I'm somewhat of a bitter realist that way. I'm glad we reconciled somewhat in his last two years, but what a waste. We all deserved better, including him.

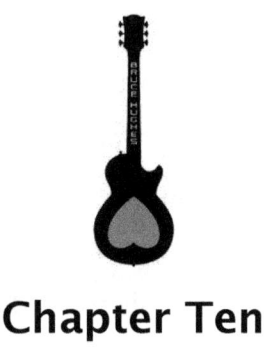

Chapter Ten

More Music

With the shock of the news barely setting in, I had to refocus, as we had another festival coming up that weekend. The Nashwaak Music Fest had finally offered us an opportunity to perform after we had unsuccessfully applied in the last three of four years. It was only a one-hour set, so we could play all original music—a first for the band, and a dream come true.

The summer had been hot and dry for weeks now, perfect weather for outdoor concerts. But when I woke the Saturday of our set, it was to a downpour.

The forecast said the rain might break around our show time, and the festival had a big, well-protected permanent stage, so we hoped we could play. There's nothing worse than a cancellation, for any reason.

We drove out late afternoon. According to radar, it looked like we could be the first act to use the mainstage that day. The production crew knew us well, warmed up the gear, took off the tarps, and said we were good to go.

Much of the crowd was gathered under two large awnings in the field to stay out of the rain showers. Being a new act, playing our own rock music at a festival that had been known more for country music than anything else was going to be interesting and satisfying, at least for the four of us on stage! We hoped it would be for the crowd too.

The boys played really well. We rocked and we rolled. The audience enjoyed it, and even a few of the other musicians were side stage watching and giving us the thumbs up. Another went so far as to lend me a guitar strap, as, for the first time since I got my Gibson electric guitar in 1983, I had forgotten mine. Lee Howe, a great guitar player well-known to this festival, graciously loaned me one of his—with his name emblazoned on it. We laugh about that whenever pictures of me wearing it surface on social media. Lee is a great guy and a much better player than I'll ever be, so if anyone really thought I was him, it was a boost.

We had a great weekend, soaking up praise from festivalgoers and music from the other bands. It felt good, another step in regaining my confidence and skills. Music heals.

A STROKE OF LUCK

A highlight that weekend was seeing my 3NE friend Sam's daughter, Michelle, with her husband, Calvin. Calvin was there as part of a really good bluegrass band and we got to hang out at their RV a couple times over the weekend. Sam would have loved it, and we all would have loved to see him there.

*

As the dog days of August wore on, I spent more time at home going for river walks with Willow, Monica sometimes joining us. It gave me time and space to reflect on the recent past and think a bit about the landmark birthday approaching. I had so much to be thankful for, but plenty of sadness as well due to so many friends and family passing of late. When I left the house, it was still just to spend time at the hospital visiting patients or rehearsing with the band.

Our band decided to make demos of a couple of songs so we could use them for digital calling cards, music festival applications, and any local or regional radio stations interested in playing us. The UnHeard shall be heard!

We decided to record live off the floor, with vocals and any lead guitar dubs added later. We rented some gear and multitalented Vaughan set up all the mics and ran the mixer during the session. He would also take them home to mix.

We picked our current favourite and show closer "High Quality" first, then the funky groove "Do You See This," which always got the crowd tapping their toes. I don't think Bob or Charles had ever done any recording, so it was an extra special day. Everyone always seems to get a bit nervous during recording sessions, but we still had fun.

A week later, Vaughan sent us the mp3s and we were pleasantly surprised how good they sounded, even with some weebles and wobbles. Two local radio stations began to play them, as did many people through Facebook and ReverbNation.

As my sixtieth birthday quickly approached, my friend Len from 95.7 The Wolf asked if we could come on his show *Blues in the Night* for a pre-taped interview introducing the songs, explaining where the band was at, and describing how I was doing on my stroke journey. It was a daytime taping and Bob and Vaughan couldn't get away from their jobs, but Charles was able to come during lunch hour to participate.

It was a blast to be back at my old station again with a bandmate, shooting the shit with another friend about music—our music. We did a couple of station ID stingers for them as well that would accompany the songs or be used in their daily rotation.

Len liked both tracks we recorded; his compliments were genuine. He knows his music and is straight up about it, friend or not. He said he couldn't wait for some more recordings, as he had his own favourites after seeing us live a couple of times over the spring and summer.

Charles and I playfully let him know we're the potatoes of the group, and that next time Bob and Vaughan, the meat, needed to be part of the interview. Their creativity steers our ship.

On my sixtieth birthday, August 22, Monica, Willow, and I stayed home rather than going out to celebrate. We listened to Len's radio show online, as we couldn't pick up the radio signal from our house. The other guys were scattered around work or home, listening when they could. Two of us had some type of online interruption and missed part of the interview, but by the time we got rebooted we got to hear the music at least. Hearing an original song on the radio never gets old. It was a nice boost for the band and a nice birthday present, too.

Three days later, though, was a sombre day. It was the second anniversary of the death of my dear friend Kris, who I wrote about earlier. Her memorial was hosted and attended by some of my oldest, closest friends since childhood, along with her husband, Roger, and son, Matt, who flew in from Calgary.

It felt good to honour her memory. We had been through junior high, high school, and university together, later reconnecting when we all moved west in that late seventies, early eighties oil boom. I quit my studies and left. She stayed and completed hers before moving to Toronto and then Calgary. We always looked out for each other; lending support any way we could. We had some wild adventures in our younger days. Mutual respect, trust, and love of life led us down many a path to find a good time or a sober second thought, whatever the occasion called for.

Later in the evening, we were all called inside the cottage by the hosts, my best friend, Ted, and his wife, Kathy, who had planted a tree last year in Kris's honour. To my utter surprise, they got me a cake and all sang "Happy Birthday" to me. My immediate reaction was to bolt, but Ted, knowing me so well, blocked my escape.

It made me very anxious. Seeing it was an awkward moment for me, after the song, Kathy told me, "Kris would have wanted to do that." I knew she was right. In fact, Kris would have loved to have sung to me in her oft-chuckled-at, off-key voice, loud and proud.

After a quick tear, I started to grin just thinking about that! Two years earlier, I barely got through playing and singing a version of Bad Company's "Seagull" at her funeral. I was honoured to have been asked to perform, and luckily, I had vocal support from a rising singing sensation, Sarah MacLoon, providing some beautiful harmony that day, as I started to choke up toward the end of the song.

I was so grateful to have something at Kris's memorial to smile about, the best way to remember a special friend like her.

A STROKE OF LUCK

*

Labour Day weekend was fast approaching, as was the band's last big show of the summer the following week, at the annual Fredericton Exhibition. The Exhibition show would be my biggest test yet, and a two-hour time slot meant I'd have to stand longer than any previous shows. That little stool I bought to keep near the side of the stage may get used yet! It also meant we'd have to bring back some of our favourite cover tunes. In the end, we decided to do a short set of covers then take a few minutes and finish with at least an hour of our music.

I was glad to see some familiar faces in the audience, including a few hospital employees who hadn't seen us perform before. You could tell they liked to rock and really enjoyed our show, taking the time to come to the stage after for a few words.

I think they were genuinely surprised how good we were and were pleased when I acknowledged them in the crowd and dedicated "Day After Day" to them, like I had done for the nurses in past shows. The long night took its toll on me, and the last three or four songs I barely hung on. Monica noticed too, saying, "It looked like you ran out of gas the last fifteen or twenty minutes." As usual, she was right!

The following week was the 2018 HJBF, and, as luck would have it, my former boss and radio station manager had a media pass for me to take in some shows, as well as to collect CDs, phone numbers, etc. for air play or interviews. I had been involved with the festival since 1992, always working, whether as a musician, stage manager, media, or emcee. This was the first time I had no such responsibilities.

I enjoyed a week of seeing whatever show interested me, along with *Blues in the Night* host Len Lynch (aka the Blues Police). We had a blast and got some good music for the station to program into rotation. The musicians really appreciated it, knowing we were the only ones who played their tracks all year round, being the local blues station, an independent able to pick what they play.

The city has five major venues and several smaller ones scattered along a few blocks of downtown Fredericton. It gave me a chance to really work my legs, going back and forth to the venues or to the car at the end of the night. By the end of the week, I was tearing up the turf almost like days of old. A pretty big difference from a year before, when we'd played the reunion show.

Recovery can come from anywhere! Len couldn't believe that in just a few days I was almost walking normally again. Stamina and fatigue were still issues, but it sure felt good to kick it almost like I used to—old school, as they say. I'm sure my gait was technically poor, but it felt good to move swiftly again, with good balance. My body and brain loved it.

*

With the annual highlight of our city done for another year (and a few days of recovery from it), it was time to focus on another opportunity to give my "50 Shades of Stay" speech to a class of occupational therapists at Eastern College in Fredericton. The director of DECH's therapeutic services, Patti, also taught part-time at the college and invited me. Of course, I accepted right away. I welcomed any opportunity to talk, inspire, and give thanks to those doing or training to do such a job. They literally are our future.

I had never been to that college before, so that day I left early to make sure I found the right building and room and to hopefully meet some of the students before my talk. My early arrival gave me just the opportunity I was hoping for—to meet the students.

With just a couple of minutes until class started, Patti arrived with a chuckle, telling me she had been down in the parking lot waiting for me. She didn't realize I'd come to town early, so she called Monica, who was home on her day off. Monica told her I had left at least an hour ago and was concerned I hadn't shown up yet. Patti told Monica she would go up to the classroom and see if I was there, and if I wasn't, she would call back.

But when Patti relayed this story to me, she forgot to tell me the part about calling her back if I *wasn't* there. I figured I would give Monica a quick call to tell her I was okay. I borrowed Patti's cellphone, and when Monica heard the phone and saw Patti's caller ID, she panicked. She assumed the worst and was in full blown tears when she picked up the phone. Once she heard my voice and I assured her I was okay, her tears subsided. Patti felt awful for her part in the misunderstanding.

In a way, I'm grateful it happened; it was such an important reminder to me that my stroke didn't affect only me. Family caregivers often suffer in silence and are left with a lot of worry and sometimes PTSD from their experiences, even when their loved ones recover well.

Once I was off the phone, Patti introduced me to the class and off I went. One of the students assisted with my presentation, clicking forward the photos as I explained each one.

They were truly interested and happy to hear from someone who had recovered with help from things they were learning to do professionally. It gave them real-life, real-time experience of what could be achieved. They were very engaged, asked good questions, and at the end posed for a photo with me and their full-sized skeleton, Fred, a classroom teaching tool. They were truly thankful for my talk and I thanked them for choosing the career they did, knowing they would help others like me well into the future.

*

The following Tuesday, on my weekly hospital visit to 3NE, another huge opportunity arose when it was confirmed I could go to the 11th World Stroke Conference in Montreal, October 17–20,

2018. I had been hoping there would be a way for me to attend the conference; it's the largest stroke-focused gathering of doctors, nurses, therapists, and researchers from all over the globe, the experts on strokes. Canada was hosting it for the first time, and I'd probably never again get the opportunity to gain such knowledge or attempt to seek answers to my unresolved questions. I'd been invited by 3NE staff, who raised the money and could only send six people total. It was the chance of a lifetime.

Having been unable to work since my strokes, finances were always an issue, but music helped pave the way, and I had tucked away money from the summer festival circuit to go toward expenses for the Montreal conference, just in case I got to go. And if I didn't?

Well, I had been trying to save for another electric guitar for many years, since I sold all others I had, so maybe I could finally get one. I needed a backup guitar, but some minor emergency always seemed to come up that required those funds. Life's like that sometimes, as I've learned too well. It was only a couple of weeks until the conference. Surely nothing else in the emergency department would pop up and I could use my tucked-away cash to go to Montreal.

All the bake sales and raffles the 3NE rehab staff held over the year paid off, and several staff were going to be able to attend. I was so happy for them and wished they all could go. Other nurses, therapists from various disciplines, and doctors from neurology and rehabilitation would be going as well to hear the latest in research, trials, best practices, and what the rest of the world is doing to deal with strokes.

It was mind boggling to think I would be sitting among them, knowing I represented their dream of success in recovery, but not knowing if it could be or had been replicated elsewhere in the world. I wasn't the only one to receive the procedure, nor a stent, but I was the world's best recovery from my type of strokes to date.

Dr. Bouma has often said to me when I start wondering why, "We got real lucky, and no one knows why." The doctors know what they did and can see the result but can't explain why it was so successful, why I lived and thrived while others die or are left seriously debilitated. I love Dr. Bouma's honesty, but as I've said before, the not knowing creates its own anxiety. She knows I can handle it and lets me lean on her a little when needed.

In order to catch the entire four-day conference, we had to leave a day early, so we all met Tuesday morning at the hospital and piled into a passenger van and headed for Montreal. Six of us: three RNs (Lisa, Julie, and Rebecca), an LPN (Heather), an OT (Steve), and me. My first road trip since my strokes.

Eight hours later, we arrived at our hotel, got unpacked, and settled in. Then we decided to go eat supper in Chinatown just beyond the hotel. We walked along, seeing many small eateries, with people lined up at most. We found a larger sit-down restaurant with a giant buffet. That was perfect for our crew, serving our appetite and budget. One of my favourite things in life is sitting having a good meal with friends, lots of laughter, and this was one of those evenings.

After we had exhausted our appetites, we thought we'd walk a few more blocks and find the giant conference centre where we would be spending the next few days. It was only a few blocks from the hotel, but we wanted to know exactly the path to the Palais des congrès de Montréal, so we knew where to go the next morning for registration.

After a mostly sleepless night, it was time to start the conference. I was really looking forward to learning more, not only about strokes but specifically about endovascular therapy, from those who had been performing the procedure from around the globe. I was interested in their results and anything they had discovered in this emerging therapy that could improve life for survivors. I also wanted to make sure I took in at least one session with each of our rehab team, to get to know better what they did and who they were as people.

We all got to choose lectures to attend. There were too many to be at them all, but we could go to enough to get a real feel for the research, trials, new technology, and stats. Day one was a blur, and at the end we met in the main lobby for a meet and greet with other delegates.

They had a nice little jazz trio, drinks, and some snacks, in a great setting. I met up with my friend Moira from the national Heart and Stroke Foundation office in Ottawa.

Moira has been so supportive of me, and a huge asset to the Heart and Stroke organization and to stroke awareness in general. It was a joy to get to know her better, as we listened to the band play some impressive numbers. Moira told me their organization was having a casual dinner and drinks session that night at another hotel and I was welcome to join them, but I was really digging the music and decided to stay, so off she went.

About twenty minutes later, she returned and said Dr. Lindsey insisted I come and meet all the rest of the team of doctors, researchers, and more. They really wanted to meet me and see for themselves this Miracle Man and his recovery. I guess seeing is believing, so I said okay and followed Moira to where the rest of her crew was gathered. I felt very honoured to be asked, especially since many of them are such well-known experts in their fields. They all had questions for me and thanked me for sharing my story. To me, sharing my story—contributing, in even a small way, to some medical research or advancement, or to giving healthcare professionals hope in their areas of expertise—is an honour.

The only thing that really shocked me that night was the price of a beer—fourteen dollars! I'm so glad I don't drink much anymore; a one-beer limit is best for obvious reasons. Having a stroke is not only hard on your health but the pocketbook, too. At those prices, staying away from it was easy.

It was getting late for me and fatigue was setting in, so I thought I should leave, even though I wanted to stay there and pick everyone's brain some more. On my way to this hotel with Moira I had been too busy talking to notice where she led us, and once I left to find my way back to our hotel, I learned something new about myself, something the strokes had affected, and something that caused me to panic slightly for the first time since I got home the previous summer.

Throughout my life I'd always had a great internal GPS, automatically knowing which direction north, south, east, and west were in. I've driven all over North America, often without a map or only a glance at one before leaving, memorizing names or directions. My sense of direction had been perfect—until now. Even though we were maybe half a dozen blocks from somewhere familiar to me, I couldn't get my brain to cooperate and send me on my way. I walked a couple of unsure blocks, and the more I thought about it the more confused I got.

Panic began to creep in, so I started looking for landmark buildings and the neon signs lit up on them that I had seen on my walk to the conference centre. At first, I didn't see anything familiar. It was a chilly fall night, I was tired, my legs weren't working well, and I knew I had limited energy, with nothing extra in the tank.

Finally, I saw a sign and building I knew were near our hotel. I made my way back toward them, then to the hotel and my room for a much-needed rest.

Something had changed in my brain that I hadn't noticed, as I hadn't been in a strange location since my strokes, always somewhere familiar. This was a new reality, from this day forward. I didn't like it at all. To this day, my internal GPS has never come back, though its absence only affects me when I'm in new or unfamiliar places.

On day two of the conference I went to more lectures and did more networking and chatting. It was fascinating to hear how other countries have set up their stroke networks and deal with patients and recoveries. For example, many African countries use cellphones to communicate and organize plans or sites for treatment, doing what they can to treat and support as many stroke patients as possible over vast areas. A patient's community plays a large role in caregiving and recovery, as do their family. They just don't have the same resources we do in Canada.

It didn't take long to see that Canada is in the top five developed countries when it comes to stroke education and support. We are so lucky, in spite of the cries of waiting lists or doctor and nursing shortages. If you have to put your life in their hands, like I did, you are going to receive good care from knowledgeable professionals and most likely live. What more could you ask for?

And you don't have a gigantic bill waiting for you when you get home.

Australia and the UK presented some interesting initiatives that caught the attention of other public healthcare system providers. The US had a lot of doctors speaking, sharing research, technology, and their medical service companies, all showing great results…for a price. When I consider the American system of private healthcare, I shudder to think how much I would owe there for having my life saved, not to mention the cost of my acute care and rehab. Monica and I would have lost most of what we owned and probably be living in our car.

I managed to attend a lecture of a Polish doctor who had three cases of stroke patients with constant legs cramps, like I had been experiencing pre- and post- stroke. After her presentation, there was a short break, so I managed to find her and ask her some questions. I asked if any of her three cases had their cramping issue resolved. She said yes, one had, but they had to remove a vertebra in the neck to do it. Not the answer I was expecting and certainly not a solution I could entertain, but I thanked her for taking the time to talk with me. At least there was a thread of an answer, although it hasn't helped with anything yet. Like my lack of GPS, the leg cramping continues to this day, and despite countless scans and examinations, no one can figure it out. In the last couple years, almost every morning when I wake up, that first little stretch on my back triggers both legs to shake violently for five to ten seconds. It's exhausting, almost like a seizure.

I also attended a session of new research reveals from Dr. Dylan Blacquiere, the doctor I'd met the previous spring at New Brunswick's stroke conference. He was a great speaker, a smart, knowledgeable guy who had left us in NB to move to Ottawa to work. Such an asset no matter where he was, in my opinion. This session also gave me a chance to sit with my nurse friend Rebecca, who also enjoyed his past talks, always looking to better educate herself with best practices.

We settled in, the lights dimmed, he started his presentation—and the first slide on the screen shocked me. He noted that just-released global data show that major stroke survivors (which I was) had a 50 percent chance of dying within five years. BAM!

I was already about a year and a half into recovery and the data floored me. I couldn't get that stat out of my head, couldn't focus on what else was being said no matter how hard I tried. I kept coming back to that statistic.

After few minutes passed, Rebecca sensed I was not okay and asked how I was doing. She knows me well, so I was honest and said that stat really rocked me. She tried to reassure me, to get me not to worry or think about it. I had beaten the toughest of odds already, and I could do it again. But I thought I may have used up all my luck the day I was saved.

A STROKE OF LUCK

This is the stuff that keeps me awake at night.

After the presentation, I stuck around hoping to talk with Dr. Blacquiere, if possible. When I had the chance, I asked why he didn't talk about this at the spring conference. I also let him know how much it rocked me. He understood how shocking it may have been and assured me this was new data, collected globally. He also was thrilled to see how far I had come in my recovery since last spring. I left the conversation feeling calmer about the statistic. (At the moment of writing this, I'm now over seven years since my strokes, so perhaps I really have missed being on the grim side of this stat as well.)

Another full day of participation left me exhausted but again thankful for the opportunity to be there. It was also nice to hear many of the delegates wish me well and say how important it is to have survivors attend and speak at these events. I wish I had the opportunity to speak at that conference. Maybe I will in the future.

Before we'd left on the trip to Montreal, I'd gotten in touch with a childhood friend, Ted Bird, who had been a well-known radio man for about the last forty years, mainly in Montreal. Whenever I visited Montreal, I always got together with Ted, staying at his place, listening to him on the radio, and just enjoying his company. He's funny and has dabbled in the comedy world. He wanted to have me on the show at the station where he now worked, to talk a bit about my story. Of course I accepted.

In my hotel room at the end of day two, I called Ted to see when would work best for him to have me on his show. He said that the next morning would be perfect. He is on a six o'clock to ten o'clock morning shift at Jewel 106.7 FM, so I could do his show and get back in time for the third day of the conference.

It was going to be a thrill to be on air with Ted. I admired his abilities, comedy, and humanity when covering news, sports, or whatever subject he addressed. I had a short run from 2005 through 2007 as a radio host of my own daily talk show in Fredericton for a small station, but this was going to be one fun interview, even if it was on a serious topic like strokes.

Now that a time and place were established, I had to come up with a plan to get there. A quick internet search on the hotel computers in the lobby gave me a map and directions, which I took back to my room to make a plan.

I could see it was a long way from our hotel to the radio station. I'd need to walk a few blocks, then take a combination of trains and buses, then walk some more to get there.

Three times I tried to embed in my head the logistics required, trying to wrap my head around what I needed to do, like I had done hundreds of times in the past. But this time was different. I just couldn't get it straight in my mind, and anxiety began to creep in—again.

I'd have to leave at 5:00 a.m. What if I got lost? Who would I call, and how, without a cellphone or the numbers of any of my travelling companions? The more I thought about it, the more it began to stress me out. The more I couldn't think it through and get a clear map in my head, the more frustrated I got, realizing another way the strokes had affected me.

After trying and trying to draw up a plan I could take with me in the morning, I gave up, completely pissed that I couldn't find the confidence to do this trip successfully or even safely. I went back to the lobby and asked about cabs and where I needed to go. The fare, they said, would be about fifty dollars. It seemed like a lot of money, but it was less than half what I saved by not going to the hockey game with other conference participants, so I booked a cab for the morning. Sure, my wallet would be lighter, but so would my anxiety.

The immediate problem was solved, but I knew this was an issue I'd have to revisit in the future.

I decided to go through the photos I shot that day. I love photography and find it helps me with my memory as well. While looking through the batch I saw a photo of me taken by another stroke survivor. There were about twenty of us at the conference, and Alon Kaplan was the first I met. We hit it off immediately. We could relate to each other's amazing journeys, but he'd taken it a step further and, after much frustration, developed his own line of rehabilitation products. He lived on his own now, in both Canada and the United States, near his children.

We met a few times during the week and that day we had lunch together. I opened my dress shirt to show him the Miracle Man T-shirt I was wearing that my sister had made me the previous Christmas. He loved it and insisted I do the Superman pose right there in the restaurant—so I did, and he snapped a photo with my camera and one with his cellphone as well. I loved how the photo turned out. We had some great discussions over those few days, and I still chat with him online from time to time.

One photo I got was of another survivor, Tom Douglas, from the United States. He was one of the best characters I met during the whole conference, so positive and helpful, always looking to improve the well-being of other stroke survivors. He told me about initiatives he was involved with in Pennsylvania, like peer support groups. He's a perfect advocate. We remain friends, again keeping in touch online.

After scrolling through my camera, I went to bed and got up at 4:00 a.m. when the alarm sounded. I took a quick shower, went downstairs for coffee and a muffin, and then took a half-hour cab ride to the Jewel 106.7 station to be on Ted and Tom's morning show.

Mile after mile, there were highways, buildings, stores, institutions, houses, and parks. I didn't really know where one community started or ended unless we crossed a river or a sign told me. The cabby was a nice guy and knew exactly where the radio station was. He even knew who Ted was, as did many locals I talked to during the week, mostly from his earlier work on the biggest stations around. So, all I had to do was sit back and enjoy the ride.

Ted met me at a door closest to their studio to let me in. It was so good to see him again, and we were both looking forward to this interview. We went into a small studio and met his on-air co-host, Tom Whelan, another well-known Montreal radio personality. After some small talk, they had to do their jobs reporting the news, traffic, sports, and their own banter before getting back to the music.

During these times we got to catch up. It felt so good to laugh with Ted again. We had both seen some hard times recently.

I'd brought Ted a box full of Monica's homemade jams, pickles, and some cookies. Anyone who has tasted any of Monica's cooking and baking knows how much he appreciated it. Of course, we got coffee and proceeded to demolish a number of cookies before we went on air. The jam and pickles would have to wait until Ted was home.

So now our time had come; we were going live after the next news update, headphones on, levels checked. Ted began: "An old friend of mine from New Brunswick, Bruce Hughes, is in the studio with me this morning. Bruce and I have known each other since elementary school and Bruce is in Montreal for a medical conference because Bruce is a medical miracle. Bruce, can you tell the medical miracle story without making me faint?"

"Well…well, I can try."

Among the chuckles, away we went. I shared my story as best I could, Ted asking good questions and us laughing at some of the answers, like my take on interviews a year earlier where I could "hear the drool running down the corner of my mouth!" Ted had his own ongoing health concerns, so we weren't flippant, but we shared an understanding of life's fragility and chose to laugh when we could.

The next few minutes flew by and we got as much of the story told as we could. Tom jumped in a couple of times with witty observations as well. It was a hoot, but also an effective, informative segment, I thought.

I stayed past my segment to chat with the two of them in between on-air time until ten o'clock. Ted felt bad about me having to spend fifty dollars on cab fare and insisted on driving me back to the hotel—but not before we ate at one of his favourite little lunch places. It gave us a chance to talk more, and we kept laughing, too.

After an awesome meal, we made the trek downtown. I wish we'd had more time, but in a half hour, we were back in front of my hotel. We both had somewhere else to be and it was a quick goodbye. Now it was time for me to get back to the conference, after a quick pit stop in my hotel.

A STROKE OF LUCK

I recognized many people from previous sessions and others from back home. Friday was a big day, honouring members, organizations, and individuals for their efforts in the field of stroke research and care. Some of the venues were huge, with good crowds to match. There were 2670 delegates from ninety-one countries, so some sessions needed the large rooms that could hold a thousand or more.

One of the people being honoured was a Brazilian doctor, Dr. Sheila Martins. She almost singlehandedly began a stroke program for the nation, starting in one hospital then branching out to five, then twenty, then twenty-five more in short order. Lives were being saved and recoveries were given a chance because of her work. Her drive and dedication were exemplary. The room exploded when she was introduced as the recipient. She was so humble in her acceptance speech, not a bit of ego, only compassion and dedication.

Another honouree was an American doctor from California, Jeffrey L. Saver M.D. I thought perhaps the L stood for Life; I saw in his bio he was considered a leading authority on endovascular therapy. He had been director of the UCLA Stroke Center since 1995. He had published something like two hundred medical papers already, where many consider twenty to thirty in a whole career to be pretty good. I noticed he was giving a talk later in the day, and I planned to attend that for sure. It would be a great opportunity to learn more about strokes in general, and possibly something respecting my personal case as well.

During the coffee break I met up with the Fredericton crew again to decide how we were going to spend our last night in the big city, and all the places we'd eat. The week had been hectic, and we wanted a night out on the town. Everyone was looking forward to it.

On my way to the afternoon sessions, I happened to see Dr. Saver. He had about fifteen minutes until his next presentation, and he was sitting alone. I took the opportunity to introduce myself and asked if he would take a couple minutes to talk with me. He graciously accepted and was blown away by my story and how I had come so far in my recovery in such a short time. He had performed procedures similar to mine, but he agreed that he had never seen anyone recover like me.

When it was time for him to get to his presentation, he apologized for having to leave and also said he thought I and other survivors should be speaking at these events. I heard that so many times throughout the conference. What an honour to meet this guy, and then have him say that! Once again, it put in perspective how lucky I must be to live to tell my tale to folks like him.

After his informative lecture, I went to another one on rehabilitation. Sitting beside me was another doctor, from Manitoba. He had developed his own aids to help a stroke patient's recovery of fine motor skills in the hands. I told him a bit about my story, so he decided to pull out some aids he had with him, mostly prototypes he used in his practice.

After I tried three or four, he claimed he couldn't seem to find any deficits in my hands, where fine motor skills are often the last to recover. I assured him there were plenty! He was shocked that only sixteen months after a series of major strokes I could use my hands, feet, and legs so well—especially my hands. He asked what I did at home to get my hands to recover so quickly.

I told him, "I'm a musician. I play guitar and write some songs." He smiled and said that was probably the best thing for me, my hands at the extremities, with the brain in between, rewiring that brain to make them perform again. Any stringed instrument or a piano, even a computer keyboard, would help get those hands and fingers moving again.

Singing was also good for the brain and important in regaining some normalcy with my speech and tone, which was not the monotone he expected from someone who'd had such severe strokes. He agreed it would be good for speech therapy. I appreciated feeling part of the solution, for actually contributing to possible future success stories by elaborating on what I did to improve my fine motor skills.

Soon my crew headed back to the hotel to get ready for our last night on the town, hoping any of the Fredericton participants who came up on their own would join us.

We decided to hit a couple of places for the evening, one a restaurant that featured chocolate in every dish. Sweet! After we assembled about a dozen of us in the hotel lobby, we headed out for what turned out to be a long walk (for me) around the city to get there, which served two purposes. One, it was a chance for more photos of the landmarks, and two, we could burn off some calories before we were about to consume a massive amount of them.

The meal and company were well worth the walk, and it all gave me another chance to get to know more about these professionals, but in a social setting. We talked about dogs, kids, music, silly things, highlights of the week, and anything else that made it to the table.

After the chocolate feast, we made our way to a small place to have some shawarma, an awesome snack of exceptionally flavourful and juicy meat, which was totally new to me. I couldn't eat much more! Then it was one more walk back to the hotel.

It was a fabulous way to wrap up the week, but I was extremely fatigued and my legs were like jelly. When we got back to the hotel, I just knew my night was going to be a long one as the leg spasms were a given at this point.

The next morning included just a couple of conference sessions. I had one more chance to hear presentations and view impressive research. I felt like a sponge, absorbing every morsel of information available.

A STROKE OF LUCK

Before leaving, I had a chance to say goodbye to the Heart and Stroke team from Ottawa who took care of my credentials and paid my conference fee. Their newsroom was somewhere I could stop in any time, all week, when I needed to rest or had some spare time to talk or get the latest daily press releases. What an incredible group of people. I saw a few familiar faces to say goodbye to or exchange email addresses or business cards with, to stay in touch in the future. My network was ballooning every day here. Then it was down the escalator for the last time and back to the hotel to pack for the ride home.

After packing, we all met with our luggage in the lobby, paid our bills, and piled back into the rented van for the journey home. Like any road trip, there was a lot of chatter at the beginning, what we liked and disliked about the week, and even more laughter, which almost seems compulsory in this group. Humour, even if it's dark, helps keep you from going crazy with worry, I think.

As the miles clicked off, some settled in for a nap or were reading, listening to the radio, checking their cellphones, and messaging loved ones they were on their way. I admired the beautiful Canadian fall scenery whizzing by.

After a couple of pit stops along the way for coffee and gas, in no time we were in Fredericton. We hugged each other as we left, but you could tell we were all looking forward to reuniting with our loved ones. I couldn't wait to see Monica and Willow!

I thanked the medical staff for including me on this epic journey, hoping they learned as much about me as I did about them. I hoped I could become the PEA they needed and deserved. I set a high bar that I was determined to reach if I wanted to be part of this incredible team.

Exhausted but riding high, I was shocked to see the state Monica was in. In fact, it was only then, over a year past my strokes, that I realized how traumatized she was. My going away had triggered an immense amount of worry and fear in her.

She was scared of a phone call in the middle of the night, someone telling her something else had happened to me—or any phone call, for that matter. She burst into tears as she told me how terrified she'd been the whole time. As I held her and told her that I was fine and would continue to be, she trembled in my arms. It was like she was unable to believe me.

I wasn't expecting it, but it was another lesson I needed to learn, and one of the reasons I wish there was more support for spouses and family member caregivers of stroke survivors. It's a legacy I have yet to fulfill but will keep pushing for, in my PEA role, speeches, and committee work.

The loved ones of stroke survivors deserve support, as well as respect and adoration for their selfless care.

Epilogue

It took me eighteen months to write this book, and another eighteen months to try to correct my many thousands of errors in the hopes of continuing to rewire my brain. My typing and spelling over this time have improved, but they both take up a great deal of energy and time.

Through all of my early recovery and even through writing this book, I've been overwhelmed with the wondering "Why?" Why did this major stroke happen to me? Why did the treatment, so untested, work on me? Why has my recovery been so good?

But after meeting all the top doctors in the world who have dealt with my type of stroke, there were no answers. Nobody knows anything more. And so, my journey to find those answers, along with this book that documents my story of pursuing them, has ended. It's time to shift my focus to living my life, and to doing what I can to help others recovering from stroke, as well as their families.

For now, these are things I know to be true:

- My life was saved by a tremendous team effort of healthcare professionals. I will forever be thankful to every one of them who helped me in my remarkable recovery.

- The quality of my life now is a direct result of sheer will, mind over matter, and hard work with the many therapists who pushed me to get better, to do what I used to do. There is no way to get around the time and effort one must put in with a never-give-up attitude, right out of the gate. The clock is ticking immediately. The need is great so must be the effort. And even if you do all this, there is no guarantee with strokes. Everyone is different, as is every recovery, but we know the results if you don't try.

- Music played a critical role in motivating me and in helping rewire my brain to function as before and to return 90 percent of my fine motor skills. I truly believe that, where possible, some form of music therapy should be built into any recovery or rehabilitation program, for stroke survivors especially. Music heals. I know it. I am living proof.

There is still much to be done to help those who find themselves having their world turned upside down by stroke. It is devastating. It can be deadly or debilitating, so when it happens, I hope they and their loved ones are lucky enough to have in their corner some of the fine healthcare professionals who saved my life and fundamentally bettered my recovery.

These professionals are the backbone of a society that can often seem broken. They are who the public are often too quick to point a finger at in a crisis, rather than lending them a hand. We all owe them our gratitude and respect, at the very least.

As I said in one of the many interviews I have done about being a "Miracle Man," I am *not* the miracle; the healthcare professionals are. I was lucky, luckier than most, to have so many in my corner and to have recovered so well.

As my friend and CBC reporter Catherine Harrop said, it was a "stroke of luck."

In my case, truer words were never spoken.

About the Author

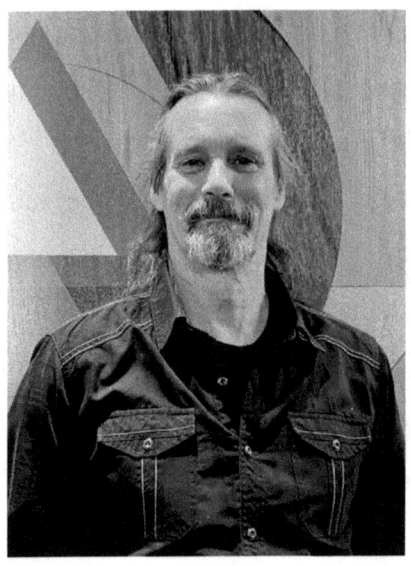

Bruce Hughes is a former educator and youth advocate with a passion for music. He plays rhythm guitar with the 70s-style rock band, The UnHeard, and is also a songwriter and singer. Bruce holds a Bachelor of Arts degree in Political Science and Psychology from the University of New Brunswick.

In May 2017, Bruce suffered a series of rare strokes that left him paralyzed from the neck down. After a miraculous recovery, Bruce now serves as the Patient Experience Advisor of Therapeutic Services at Horizon Health, where he shares his experience and provides encouragement to stroke patients and their families. He also volunteers on various committees providing perspective on patient care. Bruce currently resides in Fredericton, New Brunswick, with his wife, Monica, and their *lifesaving* dog, Willow.

Connect with Bruce on Facebook @D Bruce Hughes.

Author's Note

Thank you for taking the time to read about my stroke recovery journey. If you are a stroke survivor or a family member walking a similar path, I hope my story has brought you hope, encouragement, and a little humor along the way. Recovery is not a straight line, and it's often filled with moments of doubt and frustration—but also with unexpected victories and laughter.

I wish to extend my deepest gratitude to the medical team that gave me a second chance at life. Their dedication, skill, and compassion made all the difference. To my family, friends, and bandmates—your unwavering support and love were the fuel that kept me going even when I couldn't see the road ahead.

This book is for all of you facing life's toughest challenges. Remember: no matter how impossible things may seem, with determination, humor, and a little music, anything is possible. Stay strong, keep smiling, and never give up.

To help other readers discover my story of hope, consider posting an honest review on Amazon, Indigo and Barnes & Noble.

With sincere gratitude,
D. Bruce Hughes

www.ingramcontent.com/pod-product-compliance
Lightning Source LLC
Chambersburg PA
CBHW051546020426
42333CB00016B/2125